BRING OUT THE GLAMOUR

BRING OUT THE GLAMOUR

the air stewardess
who never was ...
and why she wasn't

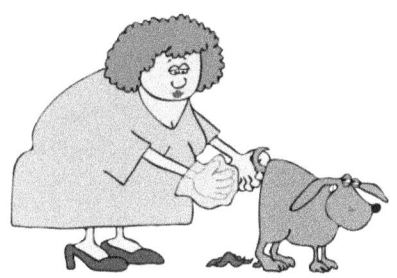

C L A U D I A   G I U L I

Giuli Publications

Giuli Publications
bringouttheglamour@gmail.com
First edition published by Giuli Publications
Copyright (c) 2012 Claudia Giuli

A catalogue record of this book is available from the British Library.

First edition 2012

ISBN: 978-0-9572061-4-4

Disclaimer:
While this book is true, in the sense of being an accurate picture of the lifestyle of cabin crew, none of the characters or the airline mentioned is real; they are a product of the author's imagination with the intention of portraying typical cabin crew and airline company personnel. Although there are real people and places referred to throughout the book, they are mingled with the fictional people and events that make up the story.

The author's target has never been any specific airline or individual, but rather to encourage people to have positive-thinking about the ability to make change in their lives by increasing one's positive self-image and overcome stigma.

Note
Part of the Royalties from this book are to be donated to support the projects of Studioo ONLUS Association (www.studioo.it). The Studioo ONLUS Association strongly believes that individuals and society as a whole can play a crucial role in promoting people's empowerment, well-being and the sustainability of the Earth's resources; this is achieved through a series of creative and social-learning processes that leverage art, culture and media to encourage a positive shift in behaviour.

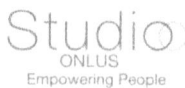

CONTENTS

ACKNOWLEDGEMENTS

A big thank you to all the people
who have shared their stories with me.

Also a huge thank you to my sister for all her support,
and to my beloved boyfriend
who has made the creation of this book possible.
Thank you, my love!

And to the wonderful world of the Internet,
for all the information with which it has empowered me.

And finally to Sam, a young Nepalese man,
for sharing with me that
'Life is busy … take it easy'

DEDICATION

I dedicate this book
to my sister Simona,
my adorable nephews
Alberto, Matteo and Francesca,
and to my partner in crimes, Alberto

Again, you can't connect the dots looking forward; you can only connect them looking backwards. So you have to trust that the dots will somehow connect in your future. You have to trust in something – your gut, destiny, life, karma, whatever. This approach has never let me down, and it has made all the difference in my life.

Steve Jobs

P R O L O G U E

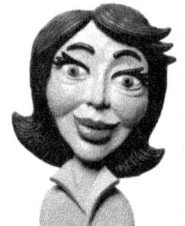'Good morning, ladies and gentleman, and welcome on board this journey into my glamorous lifestyle. Please sit back, relax and enjoy the flight and if there is anything more I can tell you to help you make your decision to become a cabin crew member, please let me know when you see me walking through the cabin one day or else crossing your path on the street. I will be very happy to tell you more stories and answer all your questions concerning this so called-glamorous job of mine.'

Now close your eyes and imagine the beautiful world of airline stewardesses and stewards. Picture them walking through the airport, wearing silvery wings and big smiles on their faces. Look how neat and well groomed they all are. Can you see them? Perfect. Look at their well-groomed hair, make-up and nails: nothing out of place, they are immaculate. Envision elegant stewardesses strutting by on high heels wearing beautiful uniforms, and gorgeous stewards walking tall with their biceps tastefully tucked into the shirts of their uniforms.

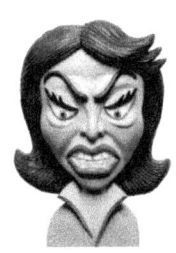Now imagine what their lives must be like. Glamorous, mysterious and fascinating. Sure! How can it be otherwise when they are flying around the world for free, getting layovers in some of the most scenic countries known to man, staying in beautiful five-star hotels paid for by the airline, and meeting interesting people? Captivating, fascinating and tempting. Sure! How can it be otherwise when they are away from their homes and husbands? Appealing, attractive, and engaging. Sure! How can it be otherwise when they have so much freedom and time on their hands?

Are you imagining all that?
Yes? Good.
Well, I am a stewardess.
What you are imagining is all crap!
Let me tell you what our lives are really like ...

ONE   I HAVE A DREAM

Hello! My name is Lilly and I just turned 24 years old a few days ago. For my birthday I went to Barbados. It is the first time I have flown in a huge plane, and also the first time I have gone to another continent. However, as sad and disappointing as it may sound – and it certainly is – what I remember most about this trip is the flight attendants. Even while on vacation, lying on a beautiful white beach and smooth sand, I could think of nothing but the flight attendants. My mind was wholly taken up with reminiscences of them. I could see them shopping at the airport's duty-free for make-up and perfume products; making their way to the aircraft while I was in the lounge waiting to board; standing in the middle of the aircraft and pointing at the doors, holding the oxygen mask and life jackets; pushing trolleys down the aisles and serving miniature cokes and spirits; securing the cabin and telling people to fasten their seat-belts; and finally waving goodbye by the doors.

How glamorous they all were! I even went further with my thoughts and imagined how I would look in one of their beautiful uniforms. Then, just as I was picturing myself wearing high heels and red lipstick, something extraordinary happened.

The same flight attendants I was imagining in my head were suddenly there before me: they were walking towards the beach. I quickly blinked my eyes a few times and pinched my skin, because I couldn't believe it was happening. As they were walking down, I was hoping and praying to have them next to me, or by me, or, worst scenario, anywhere on the beach where I could still see them.

I couldn't have been luckier that day: they took the umbrella next to mine! I promptly put my sunglasses on and watched them, stared at them and listened to them all the time. I didn't take my eyes off them. I fell in love with them. I wanted to be one of them. I dreamed to be with them right there and then. They all seemed very friendly to one another. They talked about their lives and gossiped about other people; they kissed and hugged each other; called each other 'sweetie', 'sweetheart', and 'darling'. They listened to music and sang after it. They bought colourful drinks. They went to swim together. They looked happy – and I wanted to be one of them!

As the sun was making its way to another part of the world, they all started to gather their staff and towels and headed back to their rooms, and so did I.

I followed them and stood close to them in the lift. When they pushed button 3, I pushed button 4. For the first time I could see them close-up. I studied each and every one of them carefully. They were all beautiful, even without their make-up on. And they were all of staring at me. I simply smiled at them, somehow expecting at least one of them to say something, but they didn't.

The lift reached the third floor, the doors opened and they all left, one by one. I followed them with my eyes, so wishing I was going with them but then the doors closed. When I reached my floor, I ran to my friend's room which was next to mine – oops, I haven't told you about her yet – how thoughtless of me ... Anyway, her name is Lynn and she came to Barbados with me, only to enjoy its night life, because she can't stand the sun and the heat during the day. That's all you really need to know about her.

So where was I? Oh yes, I knocked on her door.

'Lynn,' I said when she opened it, 'you have forty-five minutes to get ready and meet me downstairs at the beach bar.' (That's where the flight attendants were going to meet.) 'Tonight we are going to the GAP.' (That's where the flight attendants were all going tonight but I didn't tell her that.)

'Lilly, have you seen yourself in the mirror?' she asked

me.

'No, why?'

'Your face is the colour of a lobster and so is the rest of your body.'

'I'll be fine, Lynn, just be sure to be ready and downstairs in forty-five minutes,' I told her and walked away.

How wrong was I – so wrong that that same night I ended up in hospital with an IV attached to my arm instead, having being diagnosed with severe sunstroke! Apparently, clearly and obviously, I was so busy falling in love with the glamorous flight attendants that I completely forgot to put sunscreen lotion on and to drink water the entire six hours I was on the beach!

On my flight back home, although I was still in extreme agony, something special happened: I made friends with one of the flight attendants. She took care of me throughout the flight, giving me plenty of water to drink and making sure I took my painkillers every four hours. Then at the end of the flight she gave me a little present: a piece of paper with the following message:

Look after yourself
Love Sally

Sally@xxxxx

I gazed at her email address for a while in disbelief. Then it slowly dawned on me that I had just found a flight attendant as my friend whose name was Sally. She'd instantly become my Sally.

When I was finally home in the comfort of my bed, still recovering from the sunstroke and still in intense pain, I began to think seriously about becoming a flight attendant as I couldn't possibly just dismiss the infatuation I had just experienced with the flight attendants back in Barbados. But as I was now about to take my dream a step further, I was also fully aware that such a decision wouldn't come without obstacles. I knew for certain that my mother wouldn't easily allow me to give up on university, nor would she stand by my decision to become a flight attendant, or nevertheless would have supported me all of way through my career as an air stewardess. Needless to say, this is why I had to be highly convinced about wanting to become a flight attendant and also exceptionally cautious in making such decision.

So having spent a week collecting as much information as I possibly could on the Internet regarding becoming a flight attendant, this is what I ended up with:

⊿ *Flight attendants: job description*

The flight attendant is in charge of the cabin and responsible for the safety and comfort of the passengers: Flight attendants' primary responsibility is the safety of the aircraft cabin and its passengers. The flight attendant, being the most highly visible employee to passengers on an aircraft, must offer the most personalised service possible to each and every passenger for the entire duration of the flight.

⊿ *Flight attendants requirements: physical*

Must maintain excellent health; be well groomed; have conservative appearance; good personal hygiene; weight in proportion with height, not only to reflect the company's corporate image, but first and foremost for safety issues. A minimum height is required to reach the overhead bins. No visible tattoos, bizarre hairstyles or make-up, or body piercings are allowed.

⊿ *Flight attendants requirements: personality*

Must be poised, mature, emotionally stable, confident, outgoing and tactful, and resourceful people who can interact comfortably with strangers and remain calm under pressure. Also interpersonal skills and professionalism are of great significance.

⚐ *Flight attendants requirements: customer service*

A background in customer service is also an important consideration when applying for a flight attendant job. Must be able to handle any kind of situations dealing with the public.

⚐ *Flight attendants requirements: work hours*

Flexibility and reliability are the key words. Flights schedules and flying assignments may include weekends, nights, holidays, extended hours, overnights, and layovers.

⚐ *Flight attendants' advertisements: become a flight attendant*

- ✓ As a flight attendant, you will have a fun and exciting career that other people envy.
- ✓ As a flight attendant you and your family qualify for flight discounts to destinations throughout the world.
- ✓ The career as a flight attendant offers an exciting and privileged lifestyle that allows you to travel the world while being paid.
- ✓ Live the dream! Do you have the passion to assist people? Are you a team worker and possess leadership skills? Do you have a positive attitude? Do you like to travel? Yes? Then, what are you waiting for?

I was delighted when I realised that I fit the bill: I had all the qualifications and requirements for the job, and was ready to embark on the second part of my plan: to talk to Sally, my Sally, about being a stewardess. So I wrote her an email asking her if we could meet for coffee or lunch. Her reply left me wordless. This is what she wrote:

```
Hi Lilly, I hope you are feeling much better.
I'm going to Rome next week. Will be leaving
the 6th, a week from now, and coming back in
the evening of the day after. If you want, you
could come as my cling-on and by doing so you
will not only see what's going on behind the
curtains but I, and the other flight
attendants I will be going with, will be able
to talk to you over dinner with a nice glass
of wine in our hands. I think it'll be a good
opportunity for you to walk in our shoes for
one day. Don't worry about the hotel, you can
stay with me. What do you think? Love, Sally.
```

I had to read the email a few times. I was euphoric! I replied immediately, thanking her for the amazing opportunity that I wasn't going to miss for anything in the world.

Although I wasn't going to leave for another full week, I started to prepare my case. The weather in Rome was supposed to be nice and hot, but I packed for every possible and imaginable weather condition – rain, wind, hot days, chilly nights ... you name it.

The day before I was due to depart, while I was about to dive into the lunch I had just made for myself, I got an email from Sally. She had just sent me the flight details. In front of me were the flight number and the number of the seat I was going to occupy in the plane!

This is it, I thought, *I am going, it's real, it will happen. I will be going to Rome tomorrow with my new friend Sally, the flight attendant.*

I started to run around the kitchen table then towards my bedroom where I jumped up and down on my bed for a few times and then back to the kitchen to do it all over again. I kept running and jumping for at least ten minutes. I had never felt so elated and excited in my entire life. I was living a dream. By the time I sat down and started to eat my lunch it had gone cold, but it didn't really matter. I ate my cold spaghetti, strand by strand, daydreaming at the same time.

While eating I envisaged myself walking thorough the airport side by side with the glamorous flight attendants and the captain; checking into a five-star hotel with them; going to their favourite restaurant in Rome; ordering dinner and a nice bottle of red wine; watching people go by; asking them all sorts of questions such as the exotic places they have been to, the interesting people they have met, and the unique experiences they've had; as well as the more personal, boring questions one is supposed to ask when deciding to get a new job, such as how much money they make, how much time off they get, what are the benefits and perks, how much holiday they get, what kind of career path one can expect and so on.

Then while I was having all these lovely images in my head, I happened to catch sight of myself in the mirror. I almost fainted right then and there. My first thought was: 'How can I possibly walk side by side with them with such a messy and unfashionable haircut?' My second thought was: if I am to be one of them for one day, I must be well groomed and glamorous as well. My third and last thought was: I must do something at once. So I started to call every beauty salon in my area until I found one that would take me at once.

Thirty minutes later I was having my hair and nails done at the same time. Then another thought came to my mind: clothes. I didn't really have 'special' clothes for such a special event. So on my way back home I swung by the mall to do some shopping. I bought an evening dress to wear for dinner, a cute T-shirt to wear with jeans for a pleasant afternoon tea and two pair of shoes to match my new clothes. Then, satisfied, I went back home.

At nine o'clock at night, while I was watching TV my phone beeped. Somebody had just sent me a message. My heart stopped and I felt as if someone had impaled me on a damn skewer, as if I had suddenly turned into a shrimp!

What if the flight got cancelled? I thought. *What if Sally changed her mind or else couldn't take me with her any more?*

I pulled myself together, gathered some courage and carefully grabbed my mobile phone from on top of the kitchen table just a few metres away from where I was standing, still feeling like a shrimp. The sender was indeed Sally. Instinctively, and out of a sudden rage, I wanted to throw the phone away, or break it or set it on fire, but I didn't, I couldn't, so I squeezed it hard inside my left hand instead. I inhaled and exhaled deeply for a few times and then finally opened the message and read it.

Sally wasn't going to come to Rome because her ears were blocked due to a bad cold she'd caught during the weekend and she had to call in sick for work. However, in the message she also added that it wouldn't have made any difference to me because Penny and Charlie, two very good friends of hers, were going to operate the flight to Rome and they would take care of me just as well as she would. She also said that I would share the room at the hotel in Rome with Penny. It wasn't an ideal situation but I didn't know Sally that well either, so it really wasn't going to make much difference to me. The important thing was that I was still going. She ended the message by telling me that once at the gate, I had to make myself known to the lady behind the desk doing the boarding so that she could let Penny and Charlie know who I was at once.

On the morning of the 6th I set my alarm for eight in the morning but woke up at five without being able to fall asleep again. As I had plenty of time to get ready I spent it in the bathroom grooming myself. At eleven I was in front of the gate which was still closed because it was due to open at 11.30. I was very nervous. I took my book and started to read.

After a few failed attempts to get past the first paragraph, I closed the book and opted for my iPod instead. I kept pushing the forward button. Nothing seemed to match my mood: classical music made me want to scream; dance music made me more agitated and distressed; and blues made me sad. I quickly made a mental note to add some more music when I got back home, turned it off and went for a walk around the airport instead. I bought a few magazines and some chocolate to share with my new friends. When I went back to my gate, a few people had shown up. The gate was open now and there was a lady by the desk. As Sally instructed me, I went and introduced myself to her. She simply acknowledged it and told me to sit near by the gate, so I did.

I had just opened one of the magazines I'd just bought when I saw them coming towards my gate: two flight attendants, the Captain and the first officer. What glamour! Everybody was staring at them, me included. The Captain and the first officer wore a hat and walked together with wide steps, side by side with the same pace and their heads up. They were both tall, slim and very handsome. By the look of them they could easily be mistaken for father and son. Just behind them the two air hostesses walked side by side. Neither was very tall, and unlike the Captain and the first officer, they looked very different: one had blonde hair, tanned skin and was very slim, while the other had black hair, fair skin and was overweight. Nevertheless they were equally beautiful. Although both had ponytails, the blonde's was much longer, covering most of her back. Both wore plenty of make-up, but only the blonde had lipstick – a bright red lipstick. Their walks were also visibly different: the blonde girl walked with wide steps, just like the Captain and the first officer, whereas the brunette walked with heavy steps in a boyish manner. If I were to have guessed by the look of them, the blonde must have been Penny and the brunette Charlie.

They all walked past me and disappeared behind the doors. Shortly after, the brunette came back and stopped by the desk to talk to the woman I had given my name to earlier. The woman at the desk pointed me out and the brunette stewardess came towards me.

'Hi. You must be Lilly,' she said, and I simply nodded.

'Sally has told us all about you. We will take good care of you,' she said and then paused for a few seconds. She'd probably expected me to say something, but I had just lost the power of speech and could only nod again for I was very excited to meet her.

'My name is Penny,' she said, extending her hand to me.

I quickly did the same. This was when I was supposed to say, 'Nice to meet you, my name is Lilly,' but I didn't and nodded again instead.

'I'll see you inside then,' and off she went.

I didn't move for a while. I felt like an ice cube. Then I slowly came to my senses and started to breathe again. Everybody was watching me, wondering if I was a VIP or at least a special passenger. I stood up and went for a walk, just to relieve the tension I was feeling in my entire body. When I came back, the boarding had just started so I joined the queue. When it was my turn I took my passport and boarding pass out of my handbag. The lady checked them and off I went through the jetty. I walked through to the end of it and was now right by the plane's door where Penny was standing by, checking passengers' boarding passes. When she saw me, she welcomed me with a big smile.

'Hello, Miss Lilly, and welcome on board,' she said.

While she was talking to me, the blonde flight attendant jumped out of the flight deck and came right up to me.

'Hi, Lilly, my name is Charlie. Sally's told us all about you and your dream to become a stewardess,' then she paused for a few seconds while staring at me. As her face was close to mine, I couldn't help noticing the look on her face: an expression of compassion as if I'd just told her that my cat had died. Then she relaxed her facial muscles and put her arm around my back and took me further into the galley as she carried on talking to me.

'Listen, Lilly, we must tell you something.' They were both standing close to me, their expressions clearly quite serious. They quickly glanced at each other then Charlie started to speak again.

'Before we take you on board our fabulous life, we must tell you that once hired, you will be under the airline command and before you know it you will be selling your soul to the airline. They will plan your days and they will plan your life. They will tell you where to move and when you will be home, whether it be for one, two, four, or seven days' schedule. They will tell you who you will hang out with on your trips and where you will stay. They will also tell you what to think, what to say and what to do on a daily basis. Are you still interested in finding out more about this fabulous life of ours?'

While she was talking I was looking at her. I could see her thin lips moving, and hear her voice, which was sweet, determined yet emotionless. Her eyes were green, emerald green, beautiful, but without life. She was wearing lots of make-up, as if she had to hide some imperfection, but I couldn't find any. She was perfect. Her hair was indeed blonde but I suspected that wasn't her natural colour although there was no firm evidence as the growth of any other colour was carefully hidden away. I really didn't know what to think of her, at least for the time being.

When she finished talking she looked straight into my eyes. She was obviously waiting for me to say something as I was clearly stumbling upon my answer for a moment, but the truth was that I couldn't really understand why she was telling me such things. After all, don't all the jobs out there have some degree of discipline to follow, regulations to adhere to and supervisors to respond to? What was all the big fuss about? I thought. But since this wasn't the time nor place to start an argument or ask any questions, I simply replied as follows.

'I certainly am! I don't mind working nights, weekends and holiday seasons, nor being far away from my home. And I also love the idea of working with new people all the time.'

But little did I know back then that what Charlie was really trying to tell me was that stewardesses' well-advertised 'glamorous lifestyle' turns the majority into automatons: they become lifeless, apathetic, totally lacking in independent judgement as time goes on.

But let me not spoil the story. Let's go back in the galley with Charlie and Penny. Charlie was about to say something but Penny promptly interrupted her:

'Do you have any idea how hard it is to work in a confined space at 35,000 feet? We have to deal with all sorts of different people and situations and most of the times we do it with anger, unkindness and naughtiness because we are tired, dehydrated and exhausted.'

'We live a life that sounds pretty exciting,' Charlie resumed. 'We walk on a plane for hours on end, we're always travelling across time zones and constantly adjusting for jetlag, and spend most of our life stuck in a cramped metal tube in artificial light with super-dry stale air.'

'I cross more time zones than I care to remember,' Penny took over. 'As exciting as this may all seem, my body and mind are constantly and inevitably being affected by the lack of routine, crazy hours and jetlag. So what do I do to cope with it? What the majority of us do: I indulge in sleeping pills (Melatonin) to make myself fall asleep during the day, and caffeine pills to fight the urge to sleep during a night flight. I work on long haul flights. My body is constantly under serious stress that with time has led to my gaining weight, lacking energy, suffering from never-ending headaches, digestive problems, insomnia, persistent earaches, memory loss and—'

'And we get paid £2.40 an hour,' Charlie jumped in. 'But we love our job, don't we, Penny. Our job allows us so much freedom. We get the chance to see fab places and stay in dream-come-true hotels. But we also hate the stress and the sleep deprivation that this job involves. It starts off gradually and then as the job goes on it engraves itself on to every inch of our body with no mercy at all.'

'And we travel the globe, don't we, Charlie?' said Penny. 'And we meet lots of different people and cultures. But we are also constantly exposing ourselves to airborne diseases as well as other health hazards associated with flying, in addition to the risk of injury from turbulence or emergency landing situations.'

'And we haven't even mentioned all the standing, walking, reaching, twisting/turning, pushing/pulling, sitting, kneeling, lifting, carrying, climbing, bending and squatting this job comes with,' Charlie added with irony.

'Now,' Charlie went on, stretching the letter 'N' – 'are you still interested in finding out more about this *glamorous* life of ours?'

I'm dazed and bewildered so I merely mumble, 'Why in hell are you telling me all this? Have you girls gone totally mad?' and then I dare to ask them, 'If this job is so bad why in hell are you still doing it?'

'That's exactly the question we were waiting to hear from you,' Charlie said. 'So now, sweetheart, go and take your seat and enjoy the flight. We'll see you again when we land in Rome.'

Penny closed the door of the plane and shortly afterwards we took off.

TWO   NIGHT STOP IN ROME

Two hours later we land in Rome. We all meet outside the airport, me, Penny, Charlie, and the flight crew – to whom, I've just realised, I haven't yet been introduced. I look at them, at each and every one of them, they're all standing in front of me: Penny is talking on her cellular, Charlie is texting someone on her cellular, the Captain is looking around, and the first officer is turning his cellular on. I'm thinking that if it weren't that they're all wearing the same clothes, one wouldn't have guessed that they all knew each other or even that they were all colleagues!

They haven't talked to me since we left the plane, but they haven't talked to each other either. I'd love to approach them and start a conversation. I have so many questions buzzing in my mind, but I don't dare ask them. As I'm looking around – I'm not sure why, but most likely to hide the feeling of embarrassment or unease I am experiencing – my eyes land on a huge billboard advertising an optical brand: **SEE THE WORLD BETTER**. While I'm staring at it, I hear my name being called out. It's Penny who is calling me from a huge coach parked just on the other side of the street.

Only then do I realise that they have all gone and I'm standing in the middle of the sidewalk by myself. I rush inside the coach and here they all are, sitting apart and far away from each other. I quickly make my way towards the back of the coach, apologising to them for making them wait. However, although visibly annoyed, they don't say anything to me nor acknowledge my excuses; they simply go back to whatever they were just doing before I interrupted them. The driver closes the doors and off we go. So I sit down and settle myself in comfortably for the ride ahead.

SEE THE WORLD BETTER. I smile at the thought of it and start looking outside the window. I've never been in

Rome, I'm thinking, and here I am in Rome.

The traffic is horrendous and very loud as people keep honking their horns and yelling at each other. Drivers drive incredibly close to other cars, passing each other with only inches to spare. They constantly cut each other up, especially at big intersections. Empty spots between cars are quickly filled in. Pure madness.

I can't help noticing how many scooters there are on the streets. It's fascinating and amusing to observe them weaving through cars. Common traffic rules don't seem to apply to them, but it looks as if they make their own street code as the majority of them are driving on the opposite side of the centre line against oncoming traffic, or not stopping at red lights, or driving on the sidewalks or across crossings along with the pedestrians. Everyone else but me and the driver is either listening to music with their eyes shut or having a nap. How sad it is, I think, to miss such a free show of pure madness!

We drive past a little open market located in the middle of a small rectangular square where only pedestrians are allowed through. It's the most picturesque market I have ever seen. The square is humming, busy with people walking through arrays of stalls selling fruit, vegetables, cheese, meat, dried fruits and beans.

We drive by little alleys, closed to cars and crowded with mostly young people. I can hear them talking and laughing. They gather in groups outside coffee places or bars, smoking and drinking, a few of them kissing and hugging. I'm getting so excited. I want to be out there and can't wait to get to the hotel, drop my case and start roaming around the city. I'm so looking forward to exploring the famous beautiful scenery, architecture and historical sites with the rest of the crew, who, as they have been here many times before, will guide me around the city, or so I assume.

The coach finally comes to a stop and parks in front of an hotel. I look outside and sure enough we're in front of a five-star hotel: the Hilton. As I'm staring at it from inside the coach, I see that the crew have already got off and are now standing on the sidewalk, waiting to pick up their cases from the belly of the coach. They've all got off the coach so quickly. *They must be excited to be here as well*, I think. I quickly get off as well and join them. While we're waiting, I notice how pedestrians walking by are looking at us and smiling, as if admiring us. I feel special, a VIP almost. I start to look at them briefly and smile back at them, as famous people do when they are under the spotlight. I really don't want to go inside just now. I want to stand here by the coach for a while longer and keep enjoying the attention I'm getting. Strangely enough, the crew don't seem to notice this attention. In fact they don't look at the people at all, nor acknowledge their presence. They are just staring at the belly of the coach, anxiously waiting to grab their respective cases. A pedestrian stops Charlie and I hear him asking her 'Airline?' But Charlie takes her case and heads inside the hotel.

'How rude,' I think, but then maybe she really didn't notice him, . So I quickly step in and answer his question instead.

'Yes sir, we work for DogTired Airline.'

He looks at me, nods and simply says 'Wahoo! Very nice, very nice!' and walks away with a big smile on his face.

Once again I feel special, and since I can't get enough of such beautiful attention, I stand on the sidewalk a little longer; but nothing happens, as pedestrians are just walking by without noticing me. Why would they? I think, the crew is all gone now. They are all inside the hotel. So I take my case, which has been standing alone on the sidewalk for God knows how long, and go inside as well.

By now they have all checked in apart from Penny who is still talking to the man behind the desk. So I go and stand by Charlie and the flight crew. I'm not really sure what I'm supposed to do, nor what is to come next, so I wait for them to say something to me. Then Penny joins us.

'Shall we meet in one hour then?' she says to the rest of the crew.

'Sure,' 'Yes,' and 'Why not?' they reply and off they all go, while I'm still standing in the same spot by my case, watching them going towards the lift.

This would be the perfect time for me to say something, to shout my presence once and for all to them, but I'm unable to because I suddenly feel too embarrassed and unable to talk or move, I just keep looking at them and pondering over what I possibly might have done to spark on them such aloof and unkind behaviour towards me.

Then I see Penny looking behind her shoulders and she says. 'C'mon, Lilly, what are you waiting for? You are coming with me. Room 1015.'

I take my case and run towards her. Once in the room Penny unpacks her case and for the first time since we arrived in Rome, she talks to me.

'I hope you've enjoyed your journey so far. Please make yourself at ease now. We have an hour before meeting the crew downstairs and going out for dinner. If you wish to take a shower, please do so now. I'll take one shortly after you. Now I need to wind down a bit and feel human again. What do you think?'

'Sure,' I say, then I try to start a conversation as the silence between us is making me uneasy. 'We drove past a nice little market on our way here. Have you ever been there? Do you think we could go there later?'

'Lilly, the only places I've ever been to here in Rome are the Irish pub around the corner and the pizza place across the street.'

'You've really never wandered around the city? Is it because you don't stay in Rome long enough?'

'No, no. I do come to Rome quite often and we do stay here longer than other places but I'm always too tired so I never do anything. For me the longer we stay somewhere the more sleep I can get because all I ever want to do is to sleeeeep!.'

I can't believe my ears! *Why in earth are you doing this job then?* I want to ask her but I don't as she seems quite content with the logic of what she's just told me. Instead I take my case and put it on top of my side of the bed and open it.

While I'm looking for my toilet bag in my case to bring with me in the bathroom, I observe Penny surreptitiously. She's still in her uniform, sitting on the couch by the window and holding a glass. She looks different than earlier. She looks much older for some reason, and sadder. I zoom in on her. She has big black bags under her eyes and wrinkles all around. *What miracles make up can do!* I think. She places her glass on the table and puts her hands on her head. She plays with her hair for a while and then removes a brown wig from her head and places it on the table. I'm shocked! She's only got a scattering of locks of brown and her hair is thin! *She's going bald!*

I don't say anything but I keep glancing at her. Three empty miniature bottles of Gin are on top of the table by her side of the bed. While she holds the glass with one hand, with the other she's massaging her foot. I can't help noticing her swollen feet and how deformed her big toes are as they're both pointing outwards. She puts her glass down on the table in front of her and grabs something out of her handbag, removes her stockings and puts a bit of cream on top of the big bone and keeps massaging her foot. Only when she puts the cream down on the table do I understand what she's up to: she is applying a cream to relief inflammation because her big toes must be hurting.

She was in pain all along but never once throughout the day let on about it, I think sadly. *How can it be possible?*

She keeps massaging her feet a bit longer, then reaches inside her handbag again and takes another cream. This time she takes her jacket, jumper and shirt off as well so that she's now wearing only her bra and puts some cream on her arms and hands. Only now do I take notice of her skin: both her arms are red as a lobster and the skin is so dry that it's cut and bleeding. Her hands are not so dry, but are very red. It looks like something a dear friend of mine has – eczema or dermatitis. She developed it because she grew intolerant to chemicals irritants used in the cleaners. In fact, as part of her job as a house cleaner, she is constantly in contact with such chemicals. I now remember that because of it, she went back to school, became a nurse instead and left the cleaning business for ever. That's how unbearable the disease had become to her.

I'm wondering why Penny has it. Maybe she's allergic to some food. So, without trying to make too much of it, just to give her the chance to ignore me if she wants to, I simply say: 'A friend of mine has the same allergy. Hers is due to chemicals irritants—'

'Mine just started a year ago and it's getting worse,' she interrupts, takes a sip of her wine and continues. 'I've seen a few dermatologists and they've all told me the same thing: "Quit flying and it'll go away."'

'So why don't you quit, Penny?' The moment I say it I realise my words came out too quickly: I've put her in a difficult spot and quickly try to rectify this. 'My friend had exactly the same problem. She went back to school, acquired the skills she needed, left her job and became a nurse.'

'Lilly, I'd love to but any attempt I make to escape this job makes escape impossible! It's a Catch 22 situation: I need money to pay for school and time and energy to study. I have neither, darling!'

'Can't you work full time and go to school at the same time? You could take the online courses and study while you are en route, couldn't you?'

'I have tried it, Lilly, but this job makes me so tired, to the point where sometimes it's even hard to find the words to speak! There are so many cabin crew members I find myself working with every day with the same problem and the reason why we all have found ourselves in this mess is because we've all decided to become cabin crew for the wrong reasons. I have been doing this job for four years now and I can see myself doing it for one more year because I don't know what might happen to my health if I stayed any longer. I already feel ten years older than I actually am.

'Goddam it! If I only knew when I first started that I was going to work as a cabin crew member for only few years, I would have fucking planned my future differently. Maybe I would have gone to university first, built some skills and had a real job, then taken a gap of a year or two while doing this job. Or who knows – maybe I would have decided to do this job later in my life, as a nice way to retire, with my finances more stable so I could have done it part time and actually enjoyed it. Who the hell knows, but what I do know is that now I have no choice, no fucking skills I can sell to do anything else than flying, my damn health is getting worse by the week, I don't have enough money to pay the rent at the end of this month, and I must find another job, but I don't know what because I have no skills to sell...'

On she goes, getting more upset by the second. She's visibly upset and acting as if she were in her own little world, forgetting that I'm still there in the room with her. So I take my toilet bag and go hide in the bathroom. I lock the door behind me and feel a sudden sense of relief. I turn the water on in the shower and let it run for a while, then brush my teeth, wash my face, get undressed and take a shower. While in the shower, I can't help feeling this sense of disappointment welling up in me, probably because I'm starting to see my dreams thwarted.

Do her words indicate some kind of mental instability or is she simply being straightforwardly honest and genuine? Either way, these words are affecting me and I'm starting to feel uneasy about the ordeal of becoming a cabin crew member. The huge billboard I saw earlier at the airport jumps up in my mind and I start to realise that I should indeed *see the world better* as maybe what looked like a perfect, ideal job isn't that after all. At the same time, though, it's also true that I'm only at the beginning of my journey and there's still lots to learn. After all, there are still lots of people who are doing this job and looking fabulous, so it can't be that bad. I turn the water off, put a towel around me and open the door.

Penny is still sitting by the window, holding her glass. There's an empty miniature bottle of white wine on the table in front of her. I recognise the wine because it's the same one I just had in the plane on my way to Rome. She looks up and notices me.

'Do you want to hear something funny, Lilly? About five years ago I broke my front tooth so the dentist put a crown to restore what was left of it. Well, a few weeks ago I was eating an apple and the crown ended up in my hands! So I called the dentist, told him what'd just happened and asked how much it'd be to fix it. Between £700 and £2000, he told me. I almost dropped dead because I had just enough money in my bank account to get by until payday, let alone having £700 to pay for the damn crown.

'But not having the money to fix it was not the only problem I had. The day after I was due to work and most terrifying, in three days' time I had a wedding to go to and not just a wedding because it was my best friend's wedding, and I was going be her maid of honour! Not bridesmaid – her *maid of honour*! For the last three months I've dedicated all my spare time to help my best friend organise her big day. I helped her make planning decisions, I supported her emotionally, I kept my phone on when I was en route, just in case she needed a shoulder to cry on ... For the past few months I happily put my own life on hold and dedicated my time to this damn wedding as if it were mine, because I knew how important it was for her, my best friend. And last but not least, in the past few months I've been on a painful diet to fit inside a beautiful dress I bought five years ago when I was slimmer !

'At first, when my tooth ended up in my hand, I didn't think much of it but when I walked into the toilet and looked at myself in the mirror, the story quickly turned ugly and hopeless. At first I didn't want to believe what I was seeing so I kept closing and opening my eyes and hoping to see something different each time, but again and again the broken fucking tooth was looking right back at me. I then tried to smile in different ways, mostly by playing with my lips and the tongue in such a way that would make the gap only a bit visible, as if it were a small one, but all I could see in the mirror was someone trying her best to look mentally challenged!

'So smiling was definitively out of the question. I stopped smiling and tried to talk instead. Although the broken tooth wasn't staring right at me, as it was less visible, my speech didn't sound normal as my tongue was repeatedly and stubbornly getting caught in the gap, which wasn't small even it was unnoticeable. But while I was talking I noticed how some words only required my mouth to extend just a little bit, making the gap not so visible. So I tried to talk again. Surprisingly enough, I discovered that I could talk without moving my lips at all by only using my tongue to do all the job. But once again it looked awkward and would definitively have attracted more attention than I actually wanted in the first place. So talking was out of the question as well.

'This is when reality started to sink in: I was about to go to my best friend's wedding as her maid of honour without being able to smile or talk! If I were going to a funeral that would have been just fine and appropriate, but I wasn't. So choosing whether to go or not to the wedding was quickly fading away because I had no choice at all! The last thing I wanted was to ruin my best friend's big day. So I picked up the phone and rang her. When she answered, all I could say was "Hi".

'"Something wrong Penny?" she asked.

'I couldn't find words to describe the situation so instead I just said, "I'm coming over to your place," and hung up on her. If I couldn't describe to her what my face had become, how ugly it had become, then surely my face would speak for me, I thought. So all I needed to do was to knock at her door, wait for her to open it and greet her with the biggest smile on my face!

'But then just when I was about to leave, I went to the toilet for one last time. I looked at myself in the mirror yet again and courageously smiled back at myself: my tooth hadn't miraculously grown back!

'Defeated, I let my head rest on my shoulder, as if to find some kind of support, and just as I was about to start crying, I suddenly had an idea about how I could get my tooth back. I took my jacket, ran out of the flat and drove to Tesco, parked the car and rushed inside the supermarket. I couldn't waste any time so I went straight to the customer service desk. There were three people queuing but I couldn't wait so I ran to the front of the queue.

'"I have a problem and it's really serious," I said to all three of them. "I need to talk to the man behind the desk at once. Do you mind if I go first?"

'Nobody dared say anything – they simply nodded their heads. And here I was, in front of the man behind the desk who held the information I desperately needed to know.

'"Hi," I said, trying to keep myself as calm as I could. "I need a super-strong glue. Where can I find it?"

'"Clue?" he said in disbelief.

'"No *glue*, superglue," I said.

'"Aisle ten," he said.

'Before he had the chance to say anything else I was already in aisle ten. I found the superglue, took three packs, quickly paid for them and left the store. I ran home, leaving the car in the Tesco car park. I opened the front door of my flat and went straight for the toilet. I picked up what remained of my broken tooth on top of the counter, filled it with superglue and fixed it to the rest of my missing tooth. I kept them together with my two fingers for five minutes. I didn't move at all, hardly daring to breathe. Then, after the longest five minutes, I carefully let my fingers go of my tooth, holding my breath while looking at it … It was in one piece.

'I touched it softly and it didn't move. I ran my tongue over it and once again it didn't move. For the following hour I kept my mouth open to avoid the lower teeth touching the upper ones and at night I placed two big cotton pads inside my mouth on each side.'

Incredulous, astonished, I interrupt her. 'But superglue is a toxic substance,' I say.

'Yes it is, Lilly, and sometimes I feel dizzy and have a bad taste in my mouth, but with time I've got used to it.'

'Does that mean that you're still using superglue then?'

'Yes, it's been two months now. One more month and I will go to the dentist to have it fixed properly though.'

I stand there in disbelief, not knowing what to say. It's a funny story, no doubt, but for heaven's sake, she's been intoxicating herself for quite some time, I think, which can't be that funny!

'There's another side of the story that you may find interesting and useful for your own sake and future as a member of cabin crew,' she says, more lightly. 'Would you like a glass of wine, Lilly?'

'Yes! Thank you Penny!'

'I did tell the dentist what I do for a living, in a pitiful attempt to get him on my side and allow me to maybe pay him in instalments.

'"I'm a stewardess, you know," I said to him. "I don't make lots of money."

'To which he quickly replied, "Yeah right, you people

make more money than I do!"

'Lilly,' she says firmly, looking straight into my eyes. 'I could have almost seen the expression of contempt and disdain on his face, although he was on the other side of the phone, when he said it!'

She takes another sip of her wine and resumes. 'Lilly, you want to join the airline world, become a stewardess, right?'

I sense the doubt in her voice so I simply nod and wait to see what she's getting to.

'I'm sure you've done your homework and you can tell me how much we make yearly, can't you?'

'As a matter of fact I can.' I say proudly. 'The starting salary for cabin crew is around £18,000, plus allowances. But I've also read that it is £35,000 plus allowances if one flies long hauls.'

Penny stands up and puts her hand on my shoulder. 'This is exactly why I didn't get mad at the dentist for making such a comment because he's not to blame for being so wrongly informed – or you for that matter (although you are the moment you decide to go into a career without taking the time to do some research about it) but the media and the same airlines are indeed to blame, because they deliberately feed people with inaccurate information so they are misled and deceived.

'But let me go straight to the point that most concerns you now, Lilly, which is exactly this: forget about ever getting paid £35,000 a year. That number belongs to the past, back in the old good days of flying when contracts were made of gold, flying was the privilege of rich people and destinations were limited!

'Let's be realistic and leave the bullshit behind us for a moment and let's see what the sky is all about nowadays. The concept of flying hit the point of no return with the rising of low-cost airlines which not only drove competition through the roof but also primarily changed the entire idea of travelling. Then, as if this was not bad enough, the airline industry had yet another bigger challenge to face: the global financial crisis which hit businesses around the world so hard – and consequently the airline industry – that it forced them to their knees or, worse, pushed them out of business. As a result of which the airline industry is now facing ever more ruthless competition and turmoil within itself.

'It's no wonder then that airlines are now offering new contracts for recruits like you, Lilly, if you ever decide to become a stewardess. This is the reality that you, I and anyone who wants to be involved with the airline industry, must face. The contracts that the airline is now offering to new recruits are not much different from the one I'm on, yet they are different enough to make the new contract even worse than mine because it's rooting out generous allowance schemes and introducing instead an hourly pay scheme. In other words new recruits will take home even less money than I do and work more than I do.

'Having said this, Lilly, all you must really get into your head and hold on to firmly are the following points: one, what you're realistically looking to take home is a basic salary of £11,000 and £2.40 per hour for actual flying time, *before* taxes!; two, anything else that appears any more appealing and inviting than £11,000 and £2.40 an hour, doesn't come for free; and last but never the least, anything else you hear about this job is a mere lie.'

'What about then the £18,000 salary they are advertising?' I ask her.

'The starting salary, generously speaking, is indeed about £18,000 yearly, before taxes but it also includes all the flying time you can possibly sustain in one year by getting paid £2.40 an hour! Imagine how many hours one must work to reach £7,000 on top of the basic salary of £11,000! Do the math, Lilly, and you'll get the answer. In other words, and just to make this clear once and for all, £18,000 is the most one will ever get by doing this job full time and working his or her ass off, and that's as good as it will ever get! It isn't a "starting" salary, it's *all* you're ever going to take home.' And with that she takes a big sip of her wine.

Although surprised about what she's just told me, I particularly ponder over her last statement – 'that's as good as it will ever get' as I'm wondering how it can be possible to earn the same money over the years? Every job offers a pay rise, for God's sake! She must have noticed my expression of doubt and concern because she asks me if I have any questions.

'I do Penny,' I say. 'How is it possible that £18,000 is all one will ever get, Penny? Don't you have some kind of pay rise?'

She looks at her watch. 'I'd love to keep this conversation going, Lilly, but we must meet downstairs in fifteen minutes with the rest of the crew and I'm still wearing my damn uniform and taking a shower. We can keep on talking about this later.'

'No wait Penny, I really want to know now.'

'Because this job is not a career choice any more, Lilly, but a place where one can only work for a few years and then must move on to do something else that will allow them to feel human again and have a life. Having said this, surely we get a pay rise every year Lilly, however it's so insignificant that it really doesn't make the overall salary any more appealing over the years. How can it be when they increase it by six miserable pennies?'

'I don't understand, Penny. People think you are so glamorous. I think you are glamorous. So many women, me included, would love to take your place at any time, but here you are telling me that there's no money to be earned nor a career path to look forward to. Let alone how this job is clearly squeezing the life out of you and making you ill.'

'Lilly, hold this thought of yours until we get to dinner because there's still a lot you must hear from us as you're just at the beginning of your journey. Deal?'

I nod.

'In the meantime I want you to do something for me. Think of it as being an assignment, some kind of homework.'

I nod again.

'Good. Now I want you to start replacing the idea of doing this job because of its glamour with the idea that this job will only be a stepping stone to something you are aspiring to do in your life. What is it you are aspiring to, Lilly?'

'Well, to be a psychologist,' I mumble.

'Very good. Then this job could be a great opportunity for you to learn how to deal with all kinds of people and backgrounds. It could be a nice experience for you, Lilly. Now I'm really going to take a shower,' and off she goes.

While I'm waiting for her to take a shower, I finish getting ready. I pull the evening dress out of my case and lay it on the bed. Just next to it there happen to be the clothes that Penny was going to wear. There, before my eyes, I see an old and wrinkled T-shirt, some trousers with a few stains on them, a pair of socks, and some snickers. So I put my evening dress back in my case and wear a T-shirt and a pair of jeans instead. I put on some make-up and then get dressed. I then sit on the little couch by the window and finish my glass of wine while waiting for Penny to get ready and start dwelling on what she's just told me, which honestly is a lot to take in at once.

I can't really understand my assignment. *Why in hell would I ever think of being a psychologist when all I am dreaming of now is to become a stewardess?*

'All right, the salary isn't what the media has published, yet it still isn't too bad at all. I could live on it, especially because I'm still living with my parents. Certainly it wouldn't have made me rich but I'd be a fool to think it would,' I say loudly to myself. Surely she could work on her health though, I think: maybe eating a bit healthier and doing some exercise would help her.

While I am absorbed by this chain of thought, Penny comes out of the toilet. I don't think twice, and say to Penny vehemently, 'I think that it is quite a serious lie the airline is telling people. Maybe it wouldn't make so much difference for me, particularly, to expect a few thousands pounds less each year but certainly it would make a huge difference for people who have a family to support or a mortgage to pay—'

'Lilly, stop right there!' Penny interrupts me brutally. 'Have you listened at all to what I've just been telling you?'

I nod in fear.

'Then for heaven's sake do me a favour: quit blaming the airline! You, we, are solely responsible for our own decisions! What the hell do you expect from the airline or anybody else who is recruiting for new people? Certainly they won't lure people in by telling them what they don't want to hear, will they now? They will simply and realistically take the best aspects of the job and advertise it! It is up to you and to anyone who wants to become a stewardess to do their homework and fit the benefits the airline has to offer with their needs! How can anyone claim to be in touch with reality by expecting the airline to pay you £35,000 yearly nowadays knowing of the crisis in the airline industry? One must be completely oblivious to think this can ever happen!

'Please don't cry, Lilly. Come here, my dear, sit next to me. I am angry, indeed, and I'm wrongly taking it out of you. The only person around here who is really making an effort to know more about this job, who is doing the right thing by asking questions and seeing with her own eyes what this lifestyle of ours is all about! Look at me, Lilly' – and she gently takes my face in her hands and raises it – 'look at me. You are the hero here. People should take you as an example.'

She releases my face. 'The truth is that I'm really mad at myself because when I first started this job, I was basically naïve and totally out of touch with reality. There are already enough people who moan all the time, who are feeling miserable and trapped in a job that is gradually making them ill, and I am certainly no exception as someone who constantly moans about feeling miserable and trapped in such a vicious and wicked system as our airline/industry. I surely can't go back in time and diligently revise my initial decision to become a stewardess, but I can definitively prevent someone else from making the same mistakes that I did!

'Come closer, Lilly, I want to tell you a story which one day you might find helpful if you ever find yourself in the same situation as me. Because now that I can clearly see how oblivious I was when I first started to think that this job was like any other and consequently to understate the effects that such an exceptional and irregular lifestyle would have upon my day-to-day life and health, I want to share my experience with you.

'I look back at my past, Lilly, and I can see how I deliberately chose to be blind because – and I'm sure many colleagues of mine can relate to me in this, although I'm primarily speaking for myself – when I first joined the airline industry all I wanted was to wear the uniform, travel the world and be glamorous. Anything else was superfluous. All I ever heard about this job was how privileged the life was and how difficult it was to join it. Why then the need to find out more about it? The airline, in principle, was telling me about how privileged I was, and the Internet was telling me how much fun and how well paid it was.

'From the very beginning, when I found myself sitting in the room with the people who had just successfully gone through the interview and with the recruiters who had given me the opportunity to be the next glamorous cabin crew member, I naively chose to be deaf. The people who had just interviewed us, asking us all sort of questions all day long, finally relaxed and made us feel as if we were already part of the family, part of DogTired Airline. They were there before our eyes, beautiful, well groomed and wearing the very uniform that I, and each one in the room, was dreaming of wearing one day. They welcomed us. They made us feel special by saying that we had just been chosen over hundreds of applicants. I felt special, we felt special. They introduced themselves. All of them were operating cabin crew.

'Then they switched the TV on. A nice, warm music started to play and fill the room. Then they took turns in first introducing DogTired Airline, explaining the benefits of working for DogTired Airline, and finally the terms and conditions of our contract and how much our earnings were going to be. They talked about basic salary and the so-called allowances, which apparently we'd earn on top of our basic salary and while on duty. It was a totally new concept of earning money and quite confusing. The numbers were clearly printed on a 70-inch TV screen. Yet I didn't really give a damn about being paid £11,000 a year before taxes and £2.40 an hour before taxes when on duty. These numbers didn't mean anything because I knew that I was somehow going to earn good money and feel special.

'Moreover and sadly, even if they had told me that I was going to be paid £9,000 a year and £1.40 an hour, I still wouldn't have given a damn about it because all I really wanted and cared about was to become a glamorous flight attendant, just like these people in front of me; to be able to go to gorgeous shopping destinations like Nice for beautiful French linens and candles, or Milan for clothes or fashion week; or being able to go to sunny and exotic destinations like Barbados, Antigua or the Maldives for some sun and beautiful white beaches during cold, rainy, windy days in England.

'This is what I'd always heard about this job. This is what I had read on the Internet. This is what I thought this job was all about. So how was money ever to be a problem in such a beautiful, picturesque and colourful picture? Little did I know back then that such a glorious picture was only deceiving me into taking the job as a cabin crew member for the wrong reasons! Furthermore, I remained naively blind and deaf throughout the six-week-long training.

'The trainers made us aware of common problems related to flying such as jetlag, tiredness and insomnia, to name a few. They even divided us into groups and asked us to write how we would overcome these problems. However, because these words were somehow familiar and easy to relate to, we never once, at any given time during the entire training, questioned the degree of their effects on our health, or nevertheless on our daily lives.

'On the other hand it must be said that the trainers never once gave us a genuine explanation either, although they were all experienced cabin crew and had flown for over ten years. However, sadly, I know now why they didn't explain this to us: because they had grown accustomed to being tired and exhausted all the time, because unless one has flown before, it is quite hard to explain the real meaning of being tired or worse fatigued, so why the need to explain it? We wouldn't have understood it anyway.'

The phone rings and Penny quickly picks it up. 'I'm well ... coming down now, sorry darling ... It was Charlie,' she explains to me, 'she's been downstairs waiting for us for fifteen minutes! Let's go, Lilly.'

We both head for the door. 'Wait a second, Lilly, I need to take some Ibuprofen, my back is killing me.' She takes three pills, opens her mouth wide open and throws them in, then takes what is left of her glass of wine and swallows them. 'OK let's hurry up.' She closes the door behind her.

*

Once downstairs we head for the lounge bar of the hotel. Charlie is already there with a glass of red wine in front of her. They start talking about the flight they've just had and of the people they have recently worked with. They look at me and are about to say something but the waiter shows up. Penny orders a tonic water with ice and I have one too. Shortly after, the waiter comes with the drinks, puts them on the table and leaves. Charlie and Penny resume talking.

I lift my drink in the air and wait for Penny to do the same. I am about to say the word 'cheers' but I stop myself, glass still in the air, as I see in surprise that Penny has just put her glass in between her legs. She then takes a miniature bottle of gin from inside her handbag and adds it to the tonic water.

'Would you like some as well?' she asks while I'm still holding my glass up in the air. 'Surrrre,' I say. So she puts her glass in front of me and takes my glass from my hands. She puts it in between her legs under the table and pours a mini bottle of gin into it and resumes talking to Charlie.

I look at Charlie and Penny while they are talking, minding their own business and acting as if I weren't there. They look so different from each other. Although they are both out of their uniforms, Penny looks neglected and plain, whereas Charlie is just as glamorous with her civil clothes. Charlie is all about glamour, unlike Penny. Charlie's nails are covered with beautiful red nail polish while Penny's are unpainted and chewed to the bone. Moreover, Charlie is wearing a lovely dress and all her accessories – necklace, bracelet and ring – match the style and the colours of her dress, and though she wears different colours they are all in harmony with each other. Penny, on the other hand, looks like she's just come out of Primark in cheap, outdated clothes, and without a single accessory.

The way Charlie is sitting and the way she moves her hands make me think that she may have been a dancer in the past. She strikes me as being a strong woman, not afraid to speak her mind. I keep looking at her – I can't take my eyes off her though I don't know why. She is no ordinary woman, certainly, and nevertheless the typical blonde one would expect. She has a style of her own which is colourful and well thought out. Her body doesn't hold a gram of fat and her skin is well nurtured. She really takes time to look after herself without being overwhelmed by it. However, what is really striking is her eyes: they don't match anything of her persona and seem deprived of energy and vitality. She keeps staring at things as if on another planet – any planet but Earth. Yet she always manages to answer whatever Penny is saying or asking her. So what is so odd about her? I think. I can't really put my finger on it.

They both order one more drink, the same ones, and I do too. I wait for a gap in their conversation and then ask Charlie if she ever used to be a dancer.

'I used to be, indeed, when I was younger,' Charlie says and then begins to stare at things again.

'How long have you been flying?' I ask her.

'Penny and I started together four years ago,' she says.

'What did you do before?' I ask.

'It doesn't matter what I used to do before, now I'm part of the cabin crew and I love it,' Charlie says, glancing at Penny and, after a brief moment of silence between them, resumes: 'My family is very worried for me, my mum especially. She wants me to quit flying and get a real job as she and my entire family, for that matter, don't recognise me any more. All I care about now is having my nails done once a week and my hair twice a month. I used to read two or three books a week, I couldn't have enough of them, and now all I read is *Hello* Magazine and all the other gossip ones. But what is more bizarre is that I feel more of a woman now than ever before and I don't mind being like this.'

'Fucking hell, Charlie,' says Penny, 'you were such a different person when I first met you. What have they done to you! You look as if you've been lobotomised!'

'Lobotomised?!' Charlie says with an ironic tone. She pauses for a second to breathe and then carries on. 'Penny, although I'm lost, I am fully aware of being lost, I am fully aware of who I have become. This is what I want right now in my life: to be lost and not to have any responsibilities. To just care about my hair, and my nails being well done and polished. Period.'

They look at each other in silence and let the silence talk on their behalf for a few seconds.

'What about you, Penny?' then Charlie says, as to break the awkward silence between them.

'What about me?'

'Have you started university yet?'

'I've got no time not money for it.'

'Bullshit, you make time! I've just flown with a girl who has just graduated. She's now looking for a new job. Listen Penny, you must be realistic. Your health is going down the drain and quicker than you might think. You've now started to lose your hair as well.'

'Stop that, Charlie, don't you think that it's bad enough when I look at myself in the mirror? I don't need you to remind me of it.'

'Penny, seriously, if you could only see how miserable you have become, maybe you could have the strength and the courage to do something about it.'

'I don't know what to do. I have no skills, I'm trapped doing this job.'

'Nobody is trapped, Penny. Just start doing something and change your life accordingly. If you have no time to study, take some leave here and there in order to have more days off. Sure you will learn less money but I'm sure you can find something in your life that you can give up to mediate the loss. However, I'm honestly starting to think that this idea of yours of not being able to go to university and getting new skills to move on is becoming more an excuse to keep doing what you are doing to avoid the pressure of finding a new job and the fear of changing your daily routine. Because honestly, there are so many people who are doing this job and who had gone to university, so they've got the skills you go on about, yet they feel just as trapped by this job as you are.'

As they talk I grow more and more uneasy so I jump into the conversation and propose to start moving.

'Lilly I'm so sorry. You came to have a good time and here we are arguing. Let's go to dinner now and start all over again – what do you think?'

We all stand up and head outside.

'What about the flight crew?' I ask. 'Shouldn't we wait for them?'

'They are probably exhausted,' Charlie says. 'The airline works them to the very limit! So please, for our safety and that of the passengers, let them rest when they can!'

'What about if we go to the Irish pub around the corner?' Penny says.

'Not again! Let's do something different today,' says Charlie. 'I've noticed how fascinated you were, Lilly, when we went through that little market on our way to the hotel. Would you like to go there? I'm sure we can find a nice little restaurant with tables outside. It's such a nice day today.'

'What little market?' Penny asks Charlie. However, receiving no reply from Charlie she asks instead. 'Do you know how to get there, Charlie?'

'I've been there only once long time ago, but I'm sure the GPS will take us there.'

'Charlie, how expensive ...'

'Stop moaning, Penny, for heaven's sake. I'm sure it'll be just fine. Let's show Lilly the good side of our job, shall we? And besides it won't do any harm to remind ourselves about it either. We've got plenty of time to tell her what she's really getting to. The night is young, so let's go.'

It takes us a good three hours to get to our final destination. It could have easily taken us fifteen minutes but once we start to walk, we are immediately captivated by the beauty surrounding us and we can't resist exploring all these alleys, squares and monuments. Charlie and I want to go and visit something in particular so Charlie turns on her GPS in her cellular, types the locations and off we go.

The first place we visit is the Trevi Fountain. Ever since I saw it in the movie *La Dolce Vita*, I promised myself that one day I would go there. The fountain is more beautiful than I could have imagined – the sight of it takes our breath away!

'There's a traditional legend that if visitors throw a coin into the fountain, their dreams come true,' I say.

'Fountains aren't magical, Lilly!' Penny says while walking away with Charlie. Nevertheless, I reach inside my pocket and take a coin. There are lots of people in front of me but I manage to go closer to the edge of the fountain. Before I toss it, I spell my dream: I want to become an air hostess. Then I throw it into the water.

The second place we visit is the Spanish Steps, which Charlie wants to visit.

What a sight it is – the biggest flight of steps I have ever seen. It's crowded with people. We find a space on the steps to sit and take turns to take pictures with the camera. Shortly after, we resume our walk towards the market. As we arrive we immediately notice that the arrays of stalls are all gone, leaving the middle of the square completely empty. However, along the perimeter there are lively restaurants, cafes and pubs. Performers and musicians are entertaining small groups all around the square and many more are waiting to perform.

We pick one of the many restaurants and sit at a table outside and order a bottle of red wine.

'I can't believe you've been to Rome so many times but never once roamed the streets,' I say to Penny, looking straight into her eyes. (What I really want to say to her is: *How fucked up you must be for not taking advantage of your time in this splendid and captivating city!*)

'I'll tell you why, Lilly,' Charlie says. 'Because she's

too busy feeling sorry for herself and moaning about her job all day and year long.' She lights her cigarette and resumes talking to Penny.

'Listen, Penny, you really need to get your shit together, I can't do it for you, babe. You seriously need to stop whining about it. It's not doing you any good and honestly I'm getting quite tired of listening to you. Try to think of something nice to say about this job for a change. Here, I'll help you out. Tell me, did you have a fun afternoon so far?'

Penny nods.

'Well then, this job can't be that bad after all, can it? Look at us! We are in Rome having dinner in the middle of this beautiful square and having a nice glass of wine; we've visited the beautiful Trevi Fountain and sat on the Spanish Steps—'

'How can you two have such a different outlook on the same job you both do?' I burst in.

They look at each other in surprise.

'I mean—'

'I know what you mean, Lilly!' Charlie says with such a firm tone that I freeze.

The waiter shows up with three huge plates of pasta, places them on the table and shortly afterwards returns with a big bowl of Parmesan cheese and a basket of warm, delicious home-made bread. We start eating the pasta and dig into the basket. For a while none of us dares to say anything. We just enjoy the food. Then Charlie pours wine into each of our empty glasses and finally breaks the silence.

'So what do you think, Penny? Why do we have such different views of our identical job?'

'They are not different, Charlie, because they can't be different: our job is undoubtedly harmful. It turns people into a bunch of depressed, stressed, and unhealthy people, like me, or into hypocrite people like you! Surely you can love this job, just as one can love smoking. But we all know what prize our health must pay for such loving feeling, don't we?

You are so good to look through my problems, yet you are so blind towards yours! Just because you don't have visible health side effects like mine, it doesn't mean you're not just as screwed up, miserable and unhappy. The difference is that I say out loud, while you keep it inside. So although your attitude about work might seem positive, in reality it's just as negative and fucked up as mine.'

'C'mon, Penny, be serious, you know me better than that, sweetheart. I think most of it has to do with the way we approach what we do'

'You are so full of bullshit!'

'Let me talk Penny! For instance let's consider this for a start: you feel trapped, I feel at ease; I feel content, you feel miserable; I think of this job as being a useful gap in my life and a stepping stone to something better; you feel it's the end of your existence … Have I said anything wrong? Why are you two looking at each other?'

'Earlier, when I was talking to Penny back in her room,' I say, 'she gave me some homework to do – an assignment, so to speak. That is to start replacing the idea of doing this job because of its glamour with the idea of being a stepping stone to something I'm aspiring to be in my life instead, like being a psychologist, for instance.'

Charlie puts down her fork, positions herself further back on her chair, makes herself comfortable and stares at something or someone in front of her. After having this moment of hers, she turns slowly towards Penny and says clearly to her, 'How wise is that for a thought, Penny? I wonder how anyone is able to give people such wise advice yet not be able to benefit from it themselves. Lilly,' she adds, turning to me, 'what she said is actually the wisest thought I have ever heard regarding this job, but Penny, for fuck's sake, why do you deceive yourself like this? Why are you so hard on yourself, my darling?'

Silence descends on us all.

'Why don't we order some dessert?' I suggest, to diffuse

the atmosphere.

'Let's order another bottle of wine and why not some dessert as well,' Charlie shouts out loud, as if to break the spell.

'Ice cream is very good in Italy, should we order that?' I ask them.

Charlie is the only one to answer. 'Sure, why not?'

As I order three ice creams from the waiter, Charlie excuses herself and goes to the toilet, while Penny looks pensive. So I seize the moment and ask her a few questions to clear my confused my mind.

'Penny, if I may say so and for what it's worth, you girls are very different. How can you not see it?'

'You have no idea what flying does to people! You don't know what Charlie was like before! She encourages me to look for another job, yet she does nothing to get out of it herself. Don't you think that's being a bit awkward?'

'With all due respect, she looks much healthier than you.'

'And that's exactly the problem: she looks healthy Charlie, yet she is not! This job is frying her mind! Would you believe me if I told you that she used to be a lawyer?'

'A lawyer?'

'Precisely, Lilly! A lawyer! She used to be a lawyer and here she is: a mindless and unhappy stewardess!'

'I'm sure that she could go back to being a lawyer whenever she wants to. In fact she said that this job was only a stepping stone.'

'If that was the case, I wouldn't be so worried about her.'

'I don't understand.'

'I don't think she will ever do that, Lilly. And even more, this is exactly what she's been trying to avoid – to ever go back to being a lawyer, or to do anything at all that can be related to or even come close to law.'

'Then maybe she's planning to do something else.'

'Sure, just as I and the entire fleet are planning on doing something else, yet years later we are all still doing the same damn job!'

'How is that possible? I mean, take you for instance: why are you still flying then?'

'I guess for the same reason why people keep holding on to abusive boyfriends. Why do they do it?'

'They fear to leave them and they feel trapped.'

'Exactly. The reasons are so obvious, yet you might wonder why they don't simply overcome their fears and move on. The truth is that if you were to be in their shoes you wouldn't move on either, because you would realise that to defeat one's fear, you must first know what it is that you fear.'

'Well, I must disagree with you. In fact, this is exactly why people hold on to their misery: they must reason everything!' Just as you must have a reason to move on. Isn't it enough that flying is affecting your health?'

'You don't understand. I feel trapped, just as Charlie does as well!'

'You feel trapped! Charlie, on the other hand, doesn't! She clearly said that she likes flying. How can you possibly think that she feels trapped?'

'I don't think, I know it.'

'Have you spoken to Charlie about this?'

'How can I when she says that she loves the person she has become? Besides, the situation is more complicated than you can possibly imagine!'

'How's that?'

'I have reason to believe that she feigns being content with herself. It's all a fucking pretence! But I don't have the guts to tell her this! I don't have the courage to confront her, Lilly! When I first met her she had just moved to London from Paris. We met in a coffee shop in the city and I was reading Oscar Wilde's *The Picture of Dorian Gray*.

'"Do you have any ageing pictures of yourself up in

your attic I should know about before you start killing your friends?" she said, and held out her hand to me. "My name's Charlie," she said, "and I'm an unemployed but very successful criminal lawyer. Nice to meet you."

'We bonded right away and started to meet for coffee – at first just now and again and then regularly on our days off. One of the things we loved to do in particular was going to the theatre, because after the play we would either go to a bar and treat ourselves to a nice bottle of wine while talking about the play we had just seen, or we would go to either one of our places to enact the play we had just seen while making fun of each other performances.

'Over time we grew closer and began to confide in each other. One day we were in the park and she told me how frustrating it was looking for a job and how each failed interview was bringing her down and taking its toll on her confidence that she would ever find a job as a lawyer. Back then I didn't think much of it so I simply reminded her that it was only two months since she had moved to London and it would only be a matter of time and patience before she found one. She seemed pleased by what I said.

'A week later we were supposed to meet for lunch, as we usually did every Tuesday, but she never showed up. At first, I assumed she was running a bit late and didn't think much of it, especially because I knew that she had an interview to go to just before our meeting and it was probably going so well that it was taking her longer than expected. But after half an hour I started to grow concerned: an interview couldn't possibly last more than two hours. I tried calling her on her mobile but it was switched off.

'I ordered one more glass of wine but by the time I'd finished it I was feeling quite anxious because I still hadn't heard from her. I paid my bill and went over to her place. I rang her a few times from downstairs but she didn't answer. I stood for half an hour by her building then rang again in case I had missed her going inside, but she still didn't answer. At midnight, back at home, I was just about to call the police when I heard the doorbell. I remember this moment as if it were happening right now.

'I felt a sudden race of mixed emotions coming my way. I picked up the phone and started to tremble with fear.

'"It's Charlie, I'm downstairs, can you let me in?" I ran downstairs with happiness and fuming rage. When I reached the ground floor I was ready to go off on her. I quickly opened the doorway and there she was standing in front of me. She was still wearing her working clothes but her blouse was all wrinkled and her tights were broken. She looked messy and dirty.

'I said nothing to her. I took her inside my building and gave her a big hug. We stood there and kept hugging each other for a while without saying a word. As you might imagine, although I was relieved and happy to see her, I was also terribly sad because I knew that something terrible must had happened to her.

'We took the lift and went upstairs. When we were inside my flat, we sat on the couch in silence, side by side. At first I waited for her to say something but when I realised that it wasn't going to happen, I stood up.

'"You don't have to tell me what happened if you don't want to," I told her, "but if someone is involved in this, we must call the police tonight and deal with it. I know it won't be easy but it's got to be done."

'She quickly interrupted me before I went any further, and assured me that there wasn't any need to call the police because nobody had either injured her or worse abused her. Relieved, I sat back down next to her and waited again for her to say something. But she never did.

'I took her to my bedroom and while she was getting ready to go to bed, I went in the kitchen and grabbed a glass of water and one sleeping pill to help her relax. After she took them she quietly laid down. I stood in front of her for a while and waited for her to say something. But yet again she didn't. I remember how, although neither of us was talking, the room was buzzing with unspoken words and unfamiliar, inexplicable feelings.

'I finally gave her a kiss goodnight and switched the light off. Then just as I was struggling to find my way through the dark room, Charlie called me. I quickly turned around.

'"Yes, Charlie?" I said.

'She waited a few seconds before speaking then said, "My career as a lawyer is over, Penny."

'At that moment the room stopped buzzing as if the unfamiliar, inexplicable feelings had finally found words of shame and contempt over which they could lay down and rest. "Now please leave me alone," Charlie said, "and if you really love me and care for me, don't ask me any questions and let's not talk about this ever again." And I never did.'

Charlie returns from her pit stop to the toilette and while walking towards her chair she says to Penny: 'You know I said what I said because I love you and it hurts me to see you letting yourself go and giving up on life and all its wonderful opportunities.'

Then she goes back to her seat, lights another cigarette and starts staring at something or someone in front of her without saying anything else.

'I'm tired, Charlie,' says Penny. 'I'm always tired. I have no energy left to do anything any more. I can't think properly, I can't remember what I've eaten just yesterday, I can't dream anymore—'

'For fuck's sake, sweetheart, stop right there!' Charlie says. The pitch of her voice is so linear and unvaried that it takes us both a moment to realise what she's just said. Then she takes her glass and while holding it up on the air and just before taking it to her mouth she resumes talking again in the same tone.

'There's no doubt that something must change in your life. The routine you have created for yourself is killing you,

Penny. This is painfully obvious and unfortunately visible.'
She takes a long and seemingly joyful sip of her wine. 'Let's
suppose for one moment that you really want to put an end to
your misery, that you do want to be happy again, that you
will find another job, that you will get your hair back and
your skin nice and soft again, that you will turn your life
around, that you will do what you say you want to do. Now,
since with all due respect you have clearly been incapable of
reaching such dreams and goals of yours on your own, it is
obvious that it is time for you to change tactics and reach out
for some help.'

Penny at this point tries to say something but Charlie
promptly says, 'Do yourself a favour and do not talk, just
listen. Tonight, Penny, you will have the chance to turn your
moaning and whining into something more productive for
you and helpful for some one like Lilly, for instance, who
maybe wants to become a stewardess. Productive for you
Penny, because tonight you will make a promise to me and
Lilly to change your life around for good! Helpful for you,
Lilly, because tonight Penny will tell you why and how she's
become the worn-down battery she is now so that if you ever
decide to join cabin crew, you won't turn out like her or join
the queue of other miserable stewardesses like her. I
understand you might be a bit confused so let's reflect on a
few points …'

She moves around her chair to sit closer to us both and
leans forward over the table. She looks straight into my eyes
and asks me, 'How would you feel, Lilly, if someone gave
you some wonderful advice on how to go about something
and only later did you realise that that very person who'd
delivered such wonderful advice to you is full of shit, that
she has done nothing in her life that could remotely resemble
her praises or good intentions, let alone having achieved
anything she's committed to in her life?'

'I would think what a waste of my time it has been to be
around such person who is full of shit,' I say.

Charlie now turns towards Penny. 'And Penny, how would you feel, giving someone advice that you cannot live up to in your day-to-day life?'

'I would feel stupid about myself and a complete hypocrite,' Penny says.

Now Charlie turns towards me again. 'Lilly, now tell me, what's the point of Penny starting to fluff around, moaning and whining about her life as a member of cabin crew, if she has done nothing in her life to change such an unpleasant situation? Wouldn't you feel almost compelled to ask her: *Why in hell then are you still doing this job Penny, if it is so bad?* Wouldn't you, Lilly?'

I stare at her wordless, so she repeats the question. 'Wouldn't you, Lilly?'

I nod and she quickly turns back to Penny. 'So Penny, this is the deal. Tonight you have two choices. One is to be a hypocrite and waste Lilly's time. Two is to grab the motivation which I'm offering you and make us a promise: you will tell Lilly and me what your plans are for the next coming years and swear to us that you will commit and stick to whatever you decide to do. What will it be Penny?'

'Well,' Penny starts to say, but Charlie stops her.

'Think carefully about it, Penny, please!'

While Penny is busy with her thoughts, Charlie and I leave the table to go and watch one of the entertainers in the main square. One of them catches our attention particularly, although the razor-blade muncher and the fire-eater performers are equally as fascinating. He must be at least sixty years old and is walking and dancing on a tightrope, wearing only his loose and visibly old yellow pants! His movements are dull yet we can't take our eyes off him. The whole act is odd and could easily be misinterpreted as a big joke, but nevertheless he is entertaining people – certainly me and Charlie, as much as the other two performers are with maybe more impressive acts. We start to video recordhim and then show it to Penny when we return to our table.

As we are all watching the video, I hear Penny saying in Charlie's ear, 'I don't want to be a hypocrite. I want to turn my life around.'

At once Charlie excuses herself and leaves. She returns shortly after, places two red envelopes on the table and calls the waiter.

'Can you please bring us two pieces of paper and one pen please?'

Neither of us ask her any questions; we're simply observing her, trying to understand what she's up to. When the waiter gives her what she's asked him for, she takes the two pieces of papers and gives them to Penny.

'My dear Penny, take the pen and write down what you have decided to do to turn your life around, how you will make it happen and when the big change will actually take place. Then take what you have written and copy it on to the other piece of paper. Take your time, we are in no rush, and tell me when you are done, darling.'

She then takes the bottle of wine and pours some wine in my glass first then hers. While she is drinking she is looking at her bright orange polished nails. Then she takes some bright orange lipstick out of her little orange handbag and puts it on her lips while holding a mirror with one hand.

'How did you get to be such close friends, you two?' I ask. 'I mean, you are such different people.'

'We might look different,' Charlie replies, 'but we are very similar, although it sounds like a bad joke now. Nevertheless, when I first met Penny, she was quite a different person from now. She was alive and full of energy that radiated all around her and affected anyone she came in contact with. She smiled all the time. She had interesting thoughts and views on life. It was a pleasure to converse with her and to spend time with her.' She pauses for a few seconds and looks at her. 'And look at her now, a useless and worn-down battery she is! How sad is that Lilly?'

'I'm done, Charlie,' says Penny, 'and so are you talking about me my darling!'

'OK then, if you're happy with it, sign and date them both and place each piece of paper inside the respective red envelope and seal them both. Then write down my name on one envelope and Lilly's in the other one and give them to us.'

Penny does exactly what she's been told to do and then we both look at Charlie, waiting for her to say something.

'Penny, when are you planning to achieve your goals?' she asks her.

'In five years' time.'

'OK ladies, to make this promise of hers more exciting for all of us, I thought that we could meet up again in five years' time here in Rome, right here at this same restaurant, and open these two envelopes when we will be together again. How does that sound?'

'Well now, I can't really get out of it, can I? I really have to do something about my life,' Penny says with a big smile.

'That's exactly the point, my dear friend!' Charlie says. 'So now let's write on our envelopes the name and the address of this restaurant and the date: our meeting will take place on 23 September 2012 at 20:00. Now let's celebrate this moment and let's get ready to bring out more glamour on the table, Penny!'

'Wait a moment,' Penny says aloud 'What about you doing the same thing? I mean, although this job isn't making you visibly and physically ill, it's still affecting you mentally. I just wish you could see that, Charlie.'

I hold my breath in anticipation of what is coming next from Penny's mouth and look at her to assure her that this is the perfect time to come clean with Charlie and that it is all right to talk about the subject so much feared from both of them, although for different reasons.

'How long do you think you can carry on being so

superficial, Charlie?' Penny asks her while quickly glancing at me. Then just as she is about to say something, she poses for a few seconds while looking straight into Charlie's eyes, and she resumes talking shortly after.

'You once told me how much you wanted to meet a smart, faithful, wealthy and charismatic man. Do you really think you will find one when you are spending most of your life inside an aeroplane? Surely it can happen, but it's rare and most likely bound to become more a fairy tale than a real story with a happy ending. Having said that, just a few years ago I flew with a girl who indeed met a passenger in the plane on our way to Barbados. It was love at first sight for them. They exchanged phone numbers and shortly after started to date. A few months ago I went to St Barts in the Caribbean for work, and here they were, both of them, going to St Barts on honeymoon and sitting in the first class cabin.

'But let's be real, Charlie, for every woman whose story ends this happily, there will be many other women left with their hearts broken and with a mere piece of paper with a few number written on it as a bitter reminder of what could have happened if he had ever replied to their messages. The only men you will meet and more likely and realistically date are those who work inside the plane with you. But since you are going for men with some kind of financial stability, you will more likely date only these people who work in one section of the plane: the flight deck. Now, as much as I love and admire these guys who fly the plane, they are hardly reliable when it comes to relationships or marriage because of the nature of the job which leaves them with plenty of opportunities to be unfaithful. So the moral of my story is simply this: if you don't want to end up with the flight deck, you better get the fuck out of the plane and find another job.'

'What the fuck are you talking about, Penny?' Charlie says, stressing every single word. 'When in hell have I ever told you that I'm looking to meet someone? I'm single and happy to be one. Have you lost your mind completely?'

Penny says nothing in her defence and an awkward silence invades our table.

'Anyhow,' Charlie says, breaking the silence, 'your story reminds me of another cabin crew member who met her Prince Charming while on duty. She was on the train on her way home from work when a passenger spotted her.'

Penny stands up and says, 'I'm going to the toilet.'

'She's acting oddly,' says Charlie after Penny leaves. 'I'm wondering whether or not she should really slow down with the wine tonight! Anyhow, where was I? Yes, a passenger spotted Chantelle in the train and read her surname from the name badge pinned on her jacket. Later he called the airline and asked them to forward his contact details to Chantelle, which they did. She contacted him, they exchanged a few emails before they finally met face to face and started dating shortly after. Two years later they got married, moved to France and had a child—'

'If I ever tell this story to my friend Alex,' breaks in Lilly who's been trying unsuccessfully to meet her Prince Charming through the online dating services for the past two years, 'she wouldn't think twice about giving up her job tomorrow and joining a cabin crew!'

'God only knows what mistake that would be!' Charlie replies ironically. 'Undoubtedly finding a man can be much easier when one travels all the time like us, but unfortunately most cabin crew romantic stories begin as fairy tales and end up in heartache. Let me tell you one such story.

'I'm by the door of the plane boarding passengers for our flight to New York when I hear people screaming from the cabin. I rush in and see my colleague Ann sharply punching a man and shouting vehemently how she regretted ever having met him; a woman cursing and pulling Ann's hair; two small children screaming their heads off; two passengers trying to tear the two women apart; and all nearby passengers shamelessly screaming blue murder. I kid you not Lilly, the cabin was pandemonium! Only after the situation had calmed down and Ann taken aside to give a detailed account of her behaviour in the cabin, did we finally learn the whole story.

'It turned out she had met the fellow she was yelling at on one of her trips the year before and had dated him ever since, not realising that he was married with two children!'

'What an awful way to tell her the truth!'

'Well, not really. It was pure coincidence Lilly! A stroke of bad luck! Because Ann was supposed to go to Orlando that morning. However, at the last minute she swapped her trip for a New York one to please a colleague who was desperately trying to go to Orlando.'

'Sad story!'

'There are even sadder stories. Like cabin crew Carmen, a young, single mother who fell in love with a Jamaican who, having lured her into thinking he was madly in love with her, started borrowing money from her. She never saw a penny of the £8000 she had wired him over their two-year relationship!'

'Please stop, Charlie! These stories are making me sick!'

'Sure! But do your friend Alex a favour and tell her to stick with the online dating services if she really wants to meet a genuine Price Charming!'

Charlie lights another cigarette and begins to stare at something or someone in front of her and says nothing. I discreetly turn around to see what it is she might be looking at but nothing catches my attention so I turn around again. Her facial expression doesn't give any hints, neither do her eyes, which makes me think that maybe she's not thinking of anything at all. Nevertheless, I wait a bit longer before breaking the silence which is making me uneasy.

'Charlie, you said earlier how this job is a useful gap in your life and a stepping stone to something better. Are you planning to do something else in your life?'

She glances at me but says nothing and takes her little

pink pocket mirror from her handbag and examines herself.

'Red wine stains my lips,' she says, taking a tissue out of her handbag and adds, 'That's why I prefer to drink white wine.'

'I ask because it would make it even more exciting if you were to seal your own envelope,' I quickly add.

She tucks her mirror back in her handbag and says firmly, 'Listen, Lilly, let's get this straight once and for all! I'm not going mad and I'm neither miserable nor unhappy. You see, Penny hates this job, therefore she can't understand how anyone can possibly love it. Well, I love it and I wouldn't trade it for anything else in the world' – then she calms down and resumes talking in a more friendly tone.

'After all, Lilly, all I really want in life is very simple and that is to look pretty, do a mindless job, and get spa treatments in some exotic places where they are cheap yet very good. Having said this, what I said earlier about this job being a stepping stone to something better was for the sake of Penny. She deserves much more from life and I will do and say whatever it takes to see her doing anything else but being a member of cabin crew.'

She pauses a few seconds and resumes. 'I can't tell you how painful it is every time she tells me about yet another health problem she has to deal with because of this damn job. To give you an idea, after only two years of flying, she grew dependent on medicine to sleep and to stay awake. Now she can't sleep or stay awake without taking them! On the third year she became dependent on painkillers to ease the constant pain in her back, feet and joints, and her headaches. She takes three to six pills of Ibuprofen a day! That same year she also suffered from severe constipation problems. Then just last year she started having problems with her teeth. She had four broken teeth of which three required the complete replacement of the tooth because they had become so weak that it wasn't possible even to put a crown on them. And this year she's just started to lose her hair and develop a nasty skin rash on her arms, as you might have already noticed.'

'Why is it that your health is not as bad as Penny's when you're doing the same job?'

'Merely because I work part time hence have enough time off in between the trips to recover from extreme exhaustion! But let us talk about this later with Penny so we can really tell you what extreme exhaustion is all about and what it does to one's body. What I can tell you now though is that I too was sick all the time when I was working full time. However, as soon as I realised how harsh the airline's sickness policy was, I decided to take the problem in my own hands and went part time before it got any worse.'

'How is it harsh?'

'Because it only takes a few instances of illness to reach the final stage of the "sickness process", when you will be told to find another job because you are not fit to fly any more. As a result of this, people are scared to call in sick; hence, although they are genuinely sick, they go to work ill and their bodies get worse and worse over time, which is what's happening to Penny.'

'It's also been happening to you, according to Penny.'

'What are you talking about, Lilly? Have I not just told you how working part time has helped my health from getting like Penny's? And have you not just asked me why my health is not as bad as Penny?'

'According to Penny it is not in fact your body that is getting worse over time but your mind, and with all due respect Charlie, if this is indeed the case, I should know about it.' I stopped myself from adding – *because even the slightest and most remote chance to ever become as fucked up as you are terrifies the hell out of me* –

Charlie is about to answer to me when Penny comes back. She gazes at her in silence as Penny sits down.

'What's happening? Have I done anything wrong?' Penny says, looking at Charlie and me in turn.

'I'm telling you what's happening,' Charlie replies in a patronising tone that causes Penny to stiffen and lose confidence. 'Just because you are a discontented, dissatisfied and despondent person, it doesn't mean that everybody else must be as well. If you cannot comprehend how a person is able to enjoy being mindless and be happy then that's your problem. So please quit telling me, and Lilly, how this job has changed me into a Barbie doll and how useless I have become to you and everybody else around me. After all, who needs help here? It's you not me, because I'm happy where I am.'

Feeling somehow responsible for what had just happened, I want to explain to Penny what I have just told Charlie that might have suddenly caused her to react in such a violent matter. But just as I'm about to speak, Charlie hushes me.

'If I were you I'd keep out of this because it's none of your business, Lilly,' Charlie says, lighting a cigarette.

Neither Penny nor I say a word. After a few minutes Charlie breaks the silence and starts talking as if nothing has just happened despite the fact that both Penny and I are visibly uneasy and moreover unable to act as indeed nothing had taken place. I wait for Penny to react but by the look on her face I know she won't. So I gently stroke Penny's hand and propose to order three shots of tequila.

'What should we toast to?' Charlie asks.

'To us and to the beautiful opportunity you girls have given me to be here in Rome.'

'Then Sally is the person we should really toast to because if it weren't for her you wouldn't be here at all. How did you meet Sally in the first place anyway?' Charlie asks me.

Just before I start telling them what happened in Barbados and how Sally had left me her email on my way back from Barbados, Charlie quickly asks the waiter to bring three shots of tequila to our table and another bottle of wine.

'If I drink any more wine I won't be able to stand up or to walk,' Penny says.

'Don't you worry, if it happens I'll carry you on my back,' Charlie replies with a big smile and hugs her. Then after a short silence she continues. 'And if you become too heavy to carry, I can always leave you on one of the staircases I'll find en route and spray our magic potion on you so you'll be sleeping like Sally until tomorrow!' she says laughing.

'Magic potion?' I ask inquisitively.

'Sure, the magic potion that we spray the cabin with before passengers come on board, so they'll all go to sleep in-flight and become adorable Sallys,' Penny says. Then, just when I am about to ask something Charlie interrupts me.

'C'mon Lilly, don't be so naïve.'

Naïve? I'm thinking. *Am I naïve because I don't know that they spray the cabin with some form of sedative, or because it is a joke?* But just as I'm about to ask Charlie the question, she completely ignores me and says, 'Now we better move on! It's getting late and we still have lots to tell you, Lilly,' then she tops our glasses with more wine and turning towards Penny she says loud and clear, 'To you, my dear, the honour to start the next chapter.'

T H R E E   B R I N G   O U T M O R E
G L A M O U R

Penny   I think that a good way to start this chapter is to let Lilly ask us some questions. So Lilly what would you like to know about our job?

Lilly   I'm so curious, how do you girls spend your time when you go to wonderful places like the Caribbean or Maldives, or Bahamas or America ...?

Penny   I get asked this question every other day and every time I lie to them and give them the answer they're expecting from a glamorous stewardess. This is my speech, Lilly, and I don't even need to rehearse it any more because I know it by heart by now: on the first day I lie on the beach all day long, relax, and enjoy a few nice, colourful cocktails; on the second day I go shopping and visit sights; and on the third I relax some more in my room first and later go out with the crew to some local restaurant in town. What else can I say? Honestly. I'm there on behalf of the company and they are going somewhere on vacation and having a good time. Do you think that they want to hear the truth? Certainly not! So let's get back to reality. Despite what most people like yourself may think, the majority of us do what it's cheaper to do while abroad in beautiful places and that is: drink ...

Charlie   ... drink

Penny	... and drink again. We buy cheap miniature spirits on board and once we're back on land we buy cheap bottles of wine from some local store near the hotel where we're staying. We then meet in someone's room, share the food we brought from the plane or maybe order some room service if we get a decent discount from the hotel and then have our little party. Or else we go to our respective rooms, put up a 'Do Not Disturb' sign outside the room and shut the door behind us and only open it again the day we're due to leave.
Charlie	To be fair, there's people who do venture in town to see sights and go shopping and go out for dinner every night and drink cocktails all day long on the beach, but they are either still living with their parents or are married to people with real jobs.
Penny	As a general rule, if we don't drink, we catch up on our sleep, rest, or simply spend time on our own. If we drink, we smoke and eat all day and night in someone's room or even on the beach.
Lilly	Let me get this straight. You girls are away from home, going to beautiful places, and all you can do is drink or sleep?
Charlie	We kid you not! Despite what most people think, our glamour ends the moment we depart from our luggage at the airport. You will find no stewardess who will disagree with me on this. We all constantly joke about it so as to maybe make it less painful! The truth is that we work our arses off, we make no money and we

are here to please the needs of passengers who are getting more and more demanding as time goes on and we have ever less time to enjoy ourselves, spend quality time with those who love us, let alone the time we spend away from home. The lifestyle could be great, nobody can deny this. Going to beautiful places, being able to relax overlooking the ocean, having drinks on a beach in the middle of the week, going shopping around the world, meeting friends on the other side of the globe – it all sounds and is very exiting when it does happen and for those of us who can afford it or have any strength left to get out of their rooms and leave their beds behind them.

Lilly   C'mon on now, ladies. It's hard to believe that you go to such beautiful places and you are not able to enjoy them because you have no money or you are too exhausted to do anything. I refuse to believe it!

Charlie   For the time being, and for argument's sake, Lilly, let's leave aside that people cannot enjoy it because they don't have any money to do so. We can come back to that later, because honestly it is not the real problem here, since one could still enjoy these beautiful places by spending no money at all, for instance by relaxing and sunbathing on a beautiful beach by the ocean and watching the birds flying by and above you. The problem is that one has no idea when one first starts a career as a flight attendant of all the drinking, bad eating habits, stress, fatigue and health problems one is about to get into, which will impair and prevent anyone from enjoying anything at all in life, let alone these beautiful places we go to. And it ain't getting any better! As I've just told you earlier, but will say it again because it reflects what the airline industry has become and is all about nowadays, as time goes by we are taking care of more and more people on board, working longer hours and getting ever less time to rest and sleep! As a result of which, we are always exhausted! Do you know what being exhausted means or feel like, Lilly?

Penny Lilly, why don't you to tell us what being fatigue means for you. Give us an example, in your own words, based on your own experience.

Lilly Well, let me see. I'm quite fatigued and tired when Friday evening comes along, after getting up early in the morning and taking busy undergrounds and trains to go to work all week long, for five days in a row. But then when I go back home on Friday, I take a nice, refreshing shower, put some comfortable clothes on, and here I am, fresh as a daisy, ready to go out on Friday night.

Penny Being tired is very different from being fatigued. You can be tired, yet still be able to drive, have a conversation with someone, be responsive, active and energetic, exactly as you've just told us. But when you're feeling fatigue, you can't do any of these things. When I'm fatigued, I turn into a lethargic, apathetic individual. Even the slightest thought of socialising automatically becomes a threat to what I want to do most, which is sleep. All of a sudden the burden of working long hours in a hazardous environment, as well as sleep deprivation, hits me like a tsunami. My entire body turns into a mass of meat and bones, over which I no longer have any control. My muscles become useless, because I have no strength left to use them at all. I feel confused, disoriented, tense, irritated, weary, depressed for all day long. All I want to do is sleep and sometimes I can't do that either, because I'm too exhausted even to fall asleep. On top of that I must face all the consequences of having been in a pressurised environment at 35,000ft for hours on end. My eyes feel sore and dry, my ears ache from the constant noise I'm exposed to for hours on end inside the plane; my entire body is swollen and my skin is dry – and feels it.

Charlie   Lilly, I can't emphasise this enough. Fatigue is one of the major problems in our work environment. Something that no member of cabin crew can or will escape from. It will happen to some degree, period. This is why anyone who wants to become a stewardess ought to fully comprehend what fatigue is and how it will affect one's body and mind, in order to deal with it and minimise its effects. I will even draw you a picture, so that you will have a visual representation of it as well. Here we go.

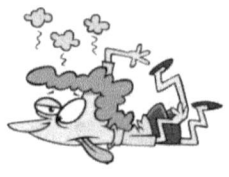

Charlie   ... But who better than you, Penny, can depict fatigue? Here you are!

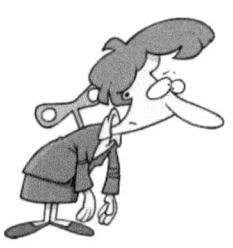

Lilly, look at these drawings! Look at these awful representations of human beings! And now imagine feeling like this every time you come back from a trip. How do you think your body, mind and soul will respond to this inevitable abuse over time?

Lilly   It's awful! Would it maybe make any difference if one worked only on short-haul trips?

Penny   The only way to ease fatigue and its awful effects on one's body, mind and soul is to work less, by working on a part-time contract. In doing so one has more time to recover from sleep deprivation and tiredness, due to the long hours of duty and not resting enough, and also from working in a hazardous environment for hours on end. Having said this the answer to your question is no, working on short-haul flights doesn't make you immune from feeling fatigue. The reasons for feeling fatigue may differ slightly, yet one's body and mind's health will still be affected just the same.

Fatigue during international flights is due mainly to flight duration and timezone differences, as well as to one's prolonged exposure to all the environmental hazards, and to the accumulation of sleep deprivation due to the busy work schedule; while on domestic/European flights fatigue is mostly related to total working hours, consecutive duty days, landing frequency, workload, duration of layovers, as well as to one's exposure to the environmental hazards and to the accumulation of sleep deprivation. However, in both cases, fatigue is mainly due to lack of rest and not enough sleep, which leads us to talk about our lovely *rest period* topic, which is another factor that compromises our ability to rest properly and consequently leads to sleep deprivation as time goes on.

Lilly   You mean a period of time before one's next trip?

Penny   Exactly so. 'Rest period' is a period of at least twelve hours from the end of one duty to the start of the next. It is designed to give us enough time to rest before our next duty. However, despite what most people might think, rest period is not the same as sleep hours, since it includes:

- time to travel to and from the airport;
- time for meals;
- time for personal hygiene;
- time to get ready for the next trip;
- time to rest;
- and finally time to go to sleep horizontally.

Charlie   Having said this, Lilly, it is very important to point out a few things that one might not take under consideration when first starting this job. First, this is not a nine to five job! Therefore, you will not commute two hours to then sit down at some desk. Your commute will only be the beginning of a long day on your feet. Second, when you come back home from work, more often than not, you won't be able to sit round a table and have supper with your husband or kids, because you won't have the energy nor desire to share such experience. All you would want to do is go to your room and shut the door behind you.

Penny   Third, the work schedule is such that one will never have enough time to rest properly, regardless of how easy the commuting might be. Having said this, although living by the airport might make the commuting less stressful and give people more time to accomplish a few of the tasks, the work schedule will affect those who live by the airport just as mercilessly as those who don't. The work schedule is what causes our fatigue, and fatigue is what depicts our own demise.

Charlie   It is time we let Lilly wear our shoes now. So let me give you an insight into what our work schedule looks like. First of all let me explain to you how our work schedule is organized. By law we have to have nine days off within our 28-day-shift schedule each month, although lately the days off have been reduced to eight. Usually and most commonly, we have a block of six days duty followed by two days off. Now let me give you an account of one of my typical six-day work schedules. I'll tell you of one in particular because it was when I finally realised that I had to work part time if I ever wanted to live longer, or else turn out like Penny or anyone else just as miserable as she is.

Penny   Keep joking about it, Charlie, if it makes you feel any better about yourself, but it won't change the truth. Your body might not be as fucked up as mine, but certainly your mind is.

Charlie   Here you go again. Tell me now if you want me to leave because if you'll say one more word about that, I swear I'll leave.

Lilly   Please can you argue about this later?

Charlie   There's nothing to talk about later Lilly. Anyhow let's move on. This was my roster: three flights to Paphos in a row, followed by a three-day trip to Orlando, Florida. My roster read:

- 22 March: short-haul trip – report at 8:30 for Paphos, Cyprus, and back in London at 20:15 the same day;

- 23 March: short-haul trip – report at 8:30 for Paphos, Cyprus, and back in London at 20:15 on the same day;
- 24 March: short-haul trip – report at 8:30 for Paphos, Cyprus, and back in London at 20:15 on the same day;
- 25 March: long-haul trip – report at 11:30 for Orlando, Florida, and back to London on 27 March at 9:30 in the morning.

Penny   Charlie, I think it'd be a good idea if we dedicate a chapter to your account. How does this title sounds like to you? Charlie's six-day work schedule.

Charlie   It sounds just fine. Let's do it.

Charlie's six-day work schedule

1st day, 22 March

The report time is at 8:30 which means that I need to be at the airport an hour earlier, so I can allow myself an hour beforehand just in case anything unforeseen happens on my way to the airport. In order for me to be at the airport by 7:30, I need to leave home at 5:50 in the morning; therefore I set my alarm clock to 5:15 am. I could sleep fifteen more minutes but I don't like to rush in the morning, so I give myself some extra time to take it easy.

So here I go. I wake up at 5:15, leave home at 5:50 sharp and catch the underground train at six o'clock. Public transportation runs smoothly today and I'm at the airport by 7:30. I relax a bit, have a cup of coffee and at 8:30 sharp I'm inside the room for my briefing. At 9:30 we take off, and four and half hours later we land at Paphos. Passengers go off, cleaners come on and half an hour later new passengers come on board. At 14:45 sharp we take off again and about five hours later we land in London. The time is now 19:45. Passengers go off, and 20 minutes later I'm outside the airport ready to go to the train station and catch my train at 20:35. By 22:00 I'm home. I hang my uniform and go and take a shower. I then put my pyjamas on, get my uniform ready for tomorrow, and go to the kitchen. While my computer is booting up, I open the fridge. I stare at it for a little bit and then take out three eggs and a bag of green salad. Can't bear to cook anything else because my whole body is sore; I'm very thirsty and exhausted. I sit down, read my emails, eat my eggs and leave the green salad behind because it smells bad (I don't dare to check the expiry date). I turn off the computer and go to sleep. It's midnight and one minute.

2nd day, 23 March

I wake up once again at 5:15 and follow the same routine of the previous day. At 5:50 I leave home. As I lock the front door, I realise that my cat is with me, outside my flat. As I'm leaning down to grab him, he runs away. So I go back home, leave the door wide open after me, and grab some cat food. I shake up the bag to make noise and here he comes. I put
some food on his bowl and run out as quickly as possible. By six o'clock and one minute too late, I'm at the underground waiting for the next train to pass, cause I have just missed the six o'clock train. Five minutes later I catch my train. Halfway through my journey the train stops. Ten minutes have gone by and the train hasn't yet moved. I try not to panic by reminding myself that I have an hour to play with. Twenty minutes later the train leaves the

station. After this the train stops briefly a few more times along the way, mainly to give other trains the right of way.

I finally arrive at the airport at 8:20. At 8:30 I'm inside the room for my briefing. As I sit down and start to relax, I feel the stress, up to now accumulated during my journey to the airport, slowly wearing off, and being quickly replaced by a feeling of tiredness instead. At 9:30 we take off, and four and half hours later we land at Paphos. Passengers go off, cleaners come on and half an hour later new passengers come on board. At 14:45 sharp we take off again and about five hours later we land in London. The time is now 19:45. Passengers go off, and 20 minutes later I'm outside the airport ready to go to the train station and catch my train.

However, on my way to the train station I get lost. Although I always take the same route to the train station from the airport, I can't remember if the train station is either on the upper floor or in a different terminal. I'm totally confused and I can't think straight. I decide to sit down and rest for five minutes, because if I start to panic about it, I will make the situation even worse and therefore more complicated to untangle. I close my eyes for ten minutes and try not to think of anything. I then open my eyes again and focus my attention on one particular thing. I choose the elevator in front of me. I then slowly expand my focus to all its proximities.

I gradually start to draw a picture of where I am. Relieved, I stand up and keep walking towards the train station but by the time I actually get to the station I have missed the 20:30 train, so now I have to take the next one at 21:00. At 21:40 I'm at the underground station. As I'm waiting for my train, a message comes through the tunnel saying that due to technical problems the next available train will arrive in twenty minutes' time.

I look around for a bench, a chair, or anything I can lean against. I see nothing, so I patiently wait and start to dream about how I will take my shoes off and leave my luggage by my front door. At last, the train arrives and it's overcrowded. I somehow manage to push myself and my luggage in. Once inside, I have people pushing me, trying to get inside as well. After a few failed attempts, the doors are eventually shut and the train can leave the platform. By 23:15 I am finally at home.

I hang up my uniform and go and take a shower. I then put my pijamas on, get my uniform ready for tomorrow, and go to the kitchen. While I'm turning my computer on, I open the fridge. I stare at it for a little bit. Nothing to eat. The only food left, which is not outdated yet, is milk. So I sit down and while I'm drinking my glass of milk I read my emails. One is coming from my sister who is planning a day out together in two days time, and another is coming from a friend of mine, who is wondering where the hell I have been and wondering why I haven't yet returned any of her phone calls yet. I attempt to reply to both of them, but unable to think straight and find any words to write, I turn off the computer instead and just before going to bed I write a note to myself and put it with my house keys. The note says: *Remember to buy a sandwich on your way home tomorrow.* Then I go to sleep. It's two o'clock in the morning.

3rd day, 24 March

I wake up once again at 5:15 and follow the same routine of the previous two days. The only difference today is that I must try to be at the underground station five minutes earlier than usual so I can have a cup of coffee because I feel quite sleepy today. At 5:55 I'm ordering my cup of coffee and a muffin to eat by the underground station and I catch the underground train at six o'clock sharp. Public transport runs smoothly today and I'm at the airport at 7:30. I relax a bit, have another cup of coffee and at 8:30 sharp I'm inside the room for my briefing. But my eyes hurt and all I can think of is going to sleep. Somehow I will get through the day, I think.

At 9:30 we take off, and four and half hours later we land in Paphos. Passengers go off, cleaners come on and half an hour later new passengers come on board. At 14:45 sharp we take off again and about five hours later we land in London. The time is now 19:45. Passengers go off, and 20 minutes later I'm outside the airport ready to go to the train station and catch my train. When I get to the train station I realise that I've been standing in front of the train time schedule's board for some time now: I have lost any sense of time and I can't figure out what time my train will depart next. Although I'm reading the time board carefully, my mind is not registering any information. So I start all over again and again and again.

After a few failed attempts I give up trying to figure it out and walk to the information desk. I tell them where I need to go and ask them to write down the platform I need to walk to and the time my train is departing. I hold the piece of paper in front of me as I walk and I finally make it: I'm inside the train, I'm safe. I sit down and set the alarm clock in my mobile to go off in thirty minutes, just two minutes before the train is due to arrive to my destination, and I fall asleep shortly after. After thirty minutes my alarm goes off and two minutes later I arrive at Victoria Station. I walk over to the underground and catch the train.

By 22:10 I'm home. I hang my uniform and go to take a long and warm shower. While I'm taking a shower I remember that I didn't buy a sandwich on my way back home. I then put my pijamas on, get my uniform ready, and prepare my luggage for my long-haul trip to Tampa the following day. So I gather a few clothes together, iron two working shirts and when I'm done I go to the kitchen. I turn my computer on and I open the fridge in the hope of magically finding some food just before my eyes. So I stare at it for a little bit but nothing happens and the fridge remains just as empty. Disappointed, I quickly close it. Nonetheless, I must find something, anything to eat. I start to open every single cabinet in the kitchen and find some biscuits in the very last one. Relieved, I go and sit down in front of my computer and eat my biscuits. I surf the Internet for a while, and when I have no biscuits left to eat, I turn off my computer. Before going to the bedroom I also write another note to myself and put it inside my pack of cigarettes. The note says: *Grocery!* I then set my alarm clock to go off at 8:15, I go to bed and switch off the light. It's 00:10.

After having tucked myself into bed, closed my eyes and secured my sleeping position, I intentionally let my mind rewind today's events so it can then play it back to me to lull me to sleep. So I gradually begin to relax and I start to experience a few free falls now and then. However, my mind tonight seems to be particularly and unusually active, hence it keeps going on and on about my day today which is making me more uneasy than sleepy. So I try to rectify my mind by changing my sleeping position. Even so, today's events now begin to mingle with yesterday's events, making my mind even more active. So I make another attempt to bring my mind to lull me and I beg *her* to stop being so damn active and unreasonably uncooperative with me tonight by imploring her to stick with today's events only and leave yesterday's ones where they belong. So I secure my sleeping position once again and close my eyes. Today's and yesterday's events now begin to mingle with random ones as well. Frustrated, I open my eyes and check the time reflected on the ceiling above my bed. I read 01:20. Although a little concerned about the passing time, I assure myself that I still have plenty of time for a good night's sleep so I optimistically secure my sleeping position once more and close my eyes.

My mind keeps stubbornly playing the same events back to me while adding new ones here and there as well. Hence I begin to toss and turn a few times before I open my eyes and courageously glance at the time on the ceiling. I read 02:05. Now, besides feeling uneasy, worried and agitated, I'm also obsessed about time and I begin to talk to myself:

I must go to sleep, I must have a good night's sleep. I must go to sleep. I'm exhausted, why can't I fall asleep? Stop thinking. Stop moving. Think of nothing. Don't move. Go to sleep. Count the sheep. Imagine them jumping a fence. 1, 2, 3 ... 56, 57, 58 ... but somehow I end up with trains in my mind instead. I begin to imagine them being delayed and I start to think of all the possible reasons why they might have been delayed. I picture a horse in front of the train, blocking it from going any farther; a person committing suicide by throwing himself in front of an oncoming train; a child accidentally pulling the manual brake, causing it to come to a complete and sudden stop; a passenger stuck between the sliding doors, preventing it from leaving.

I begin to struggle to find any more reasons. I change sleeping position once again and while doing so also realise that I haven't just lost the count of my sheep but I have been thinking of damn trains instead. I furtively look at the time on the ceiling and I read 03:32. My heartbeat spurts high instantly and I begin to despair. I lay on my back and I take hold of my head with my hands and start squeezing it hard in the hope of restraining my mind from thinking at all tonight. I start to talk to myself one again:

I must go to sleep. Stop thinking. Think of nothing. I must go to sleep. Start to count the sheep again and think only about the sheep. Only about the sheep 1, 2, 3 ... 101, 102, 103 ... but somehow I end up with roses in my mind instead. I begin to think of the meaning of the rose's colours and whether or not I would give a friend some yellow or orange roses. Yellow roses, besides being my favourite ones, stand for goodness, faith and intuition, while orange roses stand for happiness and joy. But there are also pink roses, which stand for admiration, and blue ones which stand for loyalty and wisdom. I'd say I'd give my friend a bouquet of yellow and blue roses then. But where can I find blue roses? They don't grow naturally blue. And even if I find blue ones, one can surely tell they are fake. But if I find someone who can fake them very well, maybe they'll look as natural as the red, yellow, orange and pink ones.

Why on earth am I thinking of the bloody bouquet instead of the sheep jumping the damn fence I suddenly wonder. So I change my sleeping position once more and give another quick glance at the time on the ceiling. I read 4:06. I start screaming inside my head – *This is not possible, I'm very tired, I can barely keep my eyes open, I must go to sleep, I need to sleep, I must go to sleep* – and *grouching* aloud – I must go to sleep, I must go to sleep! I've got only four hours left! – and then I keep screaming inside my head – *I must go to sleep, I must go to sleep! Go to fucking sleep, you must sleep! ...*

I grasp my duvet and pull it over my head. I let go of the duvet and bring my hand under the duvet with the rest of my body. I can feel my heartbeat. It's fast. I force myself to calm down by taking deep breaths and exhaling each of them calmly. I do this a few times before I begin to think of a stratagem to deceive my active mind and align it with my exhausted body. So I gather all the necessary weapons I need and get ready to fight. I lay on my side, secure my sleeping position and close my eyes.

I begin to think of nothing by promptly shooting and intentionally killing every thought or image that tries to lure my mind into thinking. I concentrate. I shoot and kill a few thoughts and images but somehow I end up with plants in my head instead. I begin to think of what kind of plants would survive in my flat. I need plants that don't need much sun or water. I also need a plant that is not very big either because my place is small. I like plants that have heart-shaped leaves but also diamond-shaped ones would do it.

And I like flowering plants with colourful flowers. Maybe bright yellow ones, or purple, or bright pink ones.

Why on hearth am I thinking of plants and leaves and flowers? I wonder. How in hell did I end up thinking in the first place? I wasn't supposed to think at all! So I quickly get up, grouch some more and grab a pack of cigarettes. I light one and look out of the window in despair. I imagine all the people out there who are sleeping and will shortly wake up after having had a good night's sleep. I envy them. I wish I were one of them. I glance at the clock besides me and I read 05:01, but I don't feel uneasy or apprehensive or worried any more – my mind has neutralised all of them.

Defeated, I turn the TV on and sit on the couch. I flip through the channels and find the NCIS TV programme. I pull a cover over me and start watching it. I find it difficult following the plot and wish they talked slower so I'd have time to process what they are all talking about. Nonetheless, I keep watching it, hoping to understand the plot from the images rather than from their words, but eludes me though I keep watching it motionlessly and distantly.

I hear someone knocking at my door and someone's voice. I can't tell if it's happening for real or if it's part of a dream so I ignore it. But the knocking doesn't stop – it gets louder. Someone is banging on my door, screaming my name aloud, and demanding that I switch off the alarm. Suddenly I wake up and can hear nice and clearly the banging, the yelling, and my alarm going off in my bedroom. I glance at the clock by the window. I read 8:45. I run to the bedroom and shut the alarm off. *For fuck's sake, it's been pipping loudly for the last thirty minutes* – I think. I stand still for a few seconds waiting for the man to leave. The banging and the yelling stop so I move and go to the bathroom. I quickly take a shower, get ready and I'm out of the door in only 25 minutes.

I catch the train and by 10:30 I'm at the airport. I relax a little bit, have another cup of coffee and at 11:30 sharp I'm inside the room with my colleagues for our briefing which we have every time before we operate a flight. I count the people in the room and since I am the last crew member, I close the door behind me. The person in charge of the flight glances at me and as soon as I sit down she starts the briefing.

So she introduces herself to us: her name is Ann and after having told us what she expects from us during the flight, which turned out to be what everybody else expects from us, she first gives us some specifications of the flight, such as the load, if there are any passengers with special medical needs, or deportees, infants, and so on, and then asks everyone in the room a question regarding safety procedures, including for instance the procedure we have in place if there's fire in-flight or simply about the location of certain security equipments in the plane; and a question regarding medical procedures, including the procedure we have in place for someone suffering from angina, or the location of medical equipments in the plane. These questions are mandatory before every flight, and if we don't answer them correctly, we will be offloaded and sent home on the spot.

I have a few people ahead of me, precisely five, before she will ask me the questions. I listen to the question she's asking my colleague and I try to silently answer it. My mind is racing and then goes blank. I can't answer it. I start to wonder whether or not it had been a wise choice of me to have come to work today after having had three hours of sleep last night. I feel the urge to yawn. I refrain myself from doing it.

There's a place and time for yawning, and the briefing is certainly not one of them! I say aloud in my mind. *Maybe I'm still on time to offload myself, but what do I tell her? Well, the truth, that I'm not fit to fly because I had three hours of sleep last night and I can't think, I can't focus, I feel like shit and therefore I can't possibly operate because I'd be a walking safety hazard to myself and people around me.*

But then I glance at my colleagues in my room and I quickly rectify my thoughts because they all look just as much walking hazards as me, albeit not as severely as me probably. They all have panda eyes, look miserable and unmotivated, but mostly they look annoyed, peeved and mad at themselves – most likely because they haven't called in sick this morning and done what it was best for them: remained in bed, resting their weakened bodies and restoring their strength.

Then if I am to offload myself right now there might be a great chance that they wouldn't think twice to join my cause and offload themselves as well!. Then I can't offload myself. So what should I do? Well maybe I should join their cause and look as miserable and annoyed as them. After all, if we all were to call in sick every time we are accused of exhaustion, we'd be out of work in no time. But what if an emergency is to happen today while at 35,000 feet? Will I or they be able to focus and deliver the proper procedures to fight a fire on board, or reanimate a passenger, or rescue a chocking infant? What are the procedures to fight a fire? I can't think of them. Then think harder. I inspect how bad the fire is first and then I fight it. How do I fight it though? I grab the BCF. But where is the BCF? I can't remember. Focus, damn it. I can't think. Where is the damn BCF? My mind is racing. I need to calm down, calm fucking down.

I have two people ahead of me now. My heart starts to raise. I'm cold. I can't get hold of any of my slippery thoughts inside my head. One person ahead of me. *I need to focus. I'm next. I need to pay attention to her question. Here she goes. She's looking at me. Maybe this is the right time to come clean with her. I must tell her the truth. I'm not fit to fly, damn it!*

'Where is the M5 located?'

'In the vicinity of D1L,' I jabber and keep looking at her. She says nothing so I deduct that my answer is correct.

'What medicine do you give to someone suffering from heart attack?'

'Aspirin,' I jabber again. She says nothing and moves on.

What just happened there? My answers were correct but didn't come from me. I didn't think at all, they've just come out of my mouth! I'm a robot. It shouldn't surprise me though. After all, most of the questions they ask us are always the same ones. So I've answered out of habit. That's it. Yet, I'm not fit to fly, damn it. I must tell her. I can't fly.

The briefing is over so I wait for everyone to exit the room and then I discretely approach Ann.

'Excuse me I need to have a word with you, Ann.'

'Sure darling, what is it?'

'I only had three hours of sleep last night and I don't really feel very well, maybe—'

She promptly interrupts me and says with half a smile, 'Don't we all, my dear? But don't you worry, everything will be fine because we are a team and we work as a team. C'mon now, let's go.' I'm staggered by her response but nonetheless I take my suitcase and follow her.

As I'm walking with her, my worries now focus on her. *What did she mean by 'don't we all?' Don't we all what? Have slept three hours? Or maybe that we all are tired? Or that we all don't feel well? Whatever she meant by it is not good! And worse of all, she's in charge of today's trip. This unreliable, irresponsible, dumb person is in charge and whatever she says in the next two days at 35,000 ft must be followed. She is in control and because of our chain of commands, I must obey to her.* The thought terrifies me and I stop walking.

I must offload myself. I don't feel safe with her. How can I follow such a dumb person who hasn't a clue of the implications of what she has just said to me? If anything major is to happen today, it'll be a disaster. I tell her the truth: you are too dumb and stupid and the thought of following your leadership terrifies me. I should do it! But I won't do it. OK then, I must take the problem on my hands then. I keep walking. *I'll take caffeine pills to awake my mind and my attention spam.*

From this time onwards I can't really remember much of the flight or of the trip in general as a matter of fact. However, what I do remember is the outrageous amount of caffeine pills I took in this trip to cope with my tiredness, and of sleeping pills to force myself to sleep. And also how sick, nauseated and irritable I was for the entire trip and the following few days. I must have taken at least twenty caffeine pills and six sleeping pills in only two days!

*

Charlie   Although nothing major had happened during that flight, besides the usual, such as passengers who fainted, vomited or suffered from panic attacks, when I came back to London I was determined never to find myself in that kind of hazardous situation ever again. So I began to figure out what to do and how to go about it.

The night before my flight to Orlando, I thought, I slept three hours due to insomnia, although I was extremely tired. So I began to search the Internet on how to cure tiredness, thus preventing insomnia from ever happening again. I found several recommendations which all boiled down to: sleep at least good six hours every night, eat healthily, exercise, and drink no more than one cup of coffee per day. It all sounded achievable until I looked at my roster which read the following six-day block work schedule:

- 30 March: short-haul trip – report at 8:30 for Paphos, Cyprus, and back in London at 20:15 the same day
- 31 March: short-haul trip – report at 8:00 for Thessaloniki, Greece, and back in London at 21:30 on the same day
- 1 April: short-haul trip – report at 9:30 for Sharm El Sheikh, Egypt, and back in London at 22:15 on the same day
- 2 April: long-haul trip – report at 12:00 for Tampa, Florida, and back to London on 4 April at 9:30 in the morning
- Two days off
- 7 April: short-haul trips – report at 10:00 for Nice, France, and at 17:30 for Madrid, Spain, night stop. Back to London on 8 April at 21:00
- 9 April: long-haul trip – report at 11:00 for Mali, Maldives, and back to London on 12 April at 13:00

I felt sick to my stomach when I read it! Surely, I thought, sleeping the recommended six hours tonight wouldn't be enough to feel fresh tomorrow, let alone the following working days! Moreover, eating a nice, healthy meal having been on my feet for 14 hours must be out of the question! This is when it dawned on me that I needed to work part-time if I were ever to catch up with my sleep, healthy eating habits and exercise routine. Just what you should do too, Penny!

Penny   Don't you start again. You might have found a solution to improve the health of your body, but your mind must still be dull and getting worse, even if you work part time! But please let's move on to the next question. We haven't got much time left.

Lilly   As you wish. Then my next question is: do you eat while in flight?

Charlie   I've been asked this question a few times. People must think we live on air!

Penny   They ask us that because they never see us eat. Surely not because we are a skinny bunch, Charlie!

Charlie   The question you should ask is: what do we eat in flight that makes us become so much bigger over time? To which I positively reply: it's the airline food!

Airline food is by definition recooked twice. It's cooked first in a kitchen somewhere on the ground and then reheated on the plane by us. The food is smothered in heavy sauce in a pitiful and pathetic attempt to keep it fresh and soft. It is OK if you eat it once in a blue moon, so to speak, however this is what the airline feeds us all the time while on duty at 35,000 feet, and this is who we become because of it, and turn into in our endless struggle or in our pitiful attempt to become healthier again, feel better and lose weight. Penny, pass me the pen. I want to write a little story for each one of them so you can take it home and decide which of those stewardesses you will become like one day, Lilly. Here we go.

This is the utopian stewardess and this is what she has to say for herself:

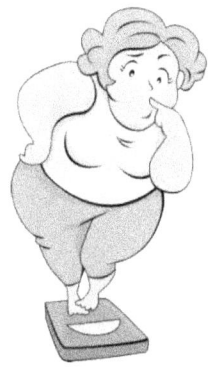

'I'm on the greatest diet in the world. I'm losing weight like nobody's business and I don't even exercise. All I do is eat everything that I can find on board, no matter what it is. The only drawback to this diet is that it doesn't work.'

This is the anorexic stewardess and this is what she has to say for herself:

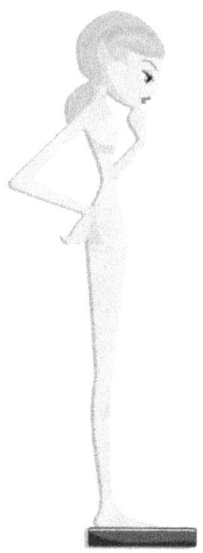

'I have lost almost ten pounds in three weeks. In one flight, five hours in duration, the most I got to eat was two bags of pretzels. The total for the pretzels grossness was only 80 calories. Plus the little pretzel bags are impossible to open and all that struggling with the bag increases my metabolism, so I get to factor that in, too. The only drawback to this diet is that I have become anorexic.'

This is the neurotic stewardess and this is what she has to say for herself:

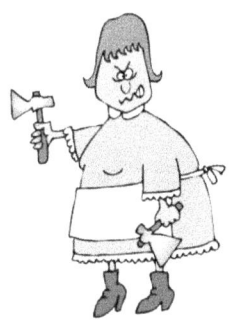

'I want to go to the gym. I want to eat healthily. I want to be healthy. The only drawback to this diet is that the 'wanting' doesn't give me a reasonable schedule to go to the gym regularly, nor the time to go to the grocery to buy healthy food! So I eat whatever I find in the plane.'

This is the frustrated stewardess and this is what she has to say for herself:

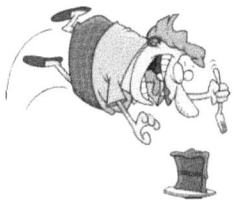

'When I work I drink lots of water, because I know that's important to keep me hydrated. I even stay away from chocolate bars and preheated airline's hot meals, because I know that's not healthy for me

either. I also eat all the fruit and vegetables I can find on board, because I know that's good for me too. The only drawback to this diet is that I get so hungry when I get off work, that I eat everything that's available to me, regardless what time of the day or night it might be.'

This is the optimistic stewardess and this is what she has to say for herself:

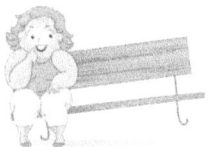

'This is my diet for the next two months. So far I have lost 20 pounds in four days: for breakfast, lunch and dinner I eat a set of foods that I cannot vary nor substitute. For example, for breakfast I eat only grapefruit and drink coffee or tea. For lunch I eat pasta with olive oil and basil, and one small apple. For dinner a steak with lettuce salad and tomato juice. The only drawback to this diet is that my work schedule is so random and the hours so crazy that most of the time I can't buy the food I need because the grocery store is shut. So I give up dieting and eat what's available in the plane.'

This is the happy stewardess and this is what she has to say for herself:

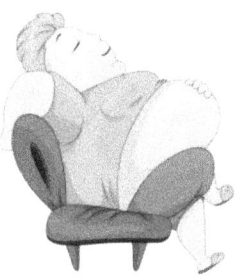

'*A few months ago I subscribed to a gym near my house. I thought I could afford to pay £30 a month for it, but I really couldn't so I cancelled the membership and stopped going. I then started to use the gyms provided by the hotels when I was en route, but I had to give that up as well because I was either too exhausted to go or felt nauseous from all the food I had eaten in the plane throughout the day. So I gave up going to the gym altogether and stopped worrying about my weight.*'

This is the nostalgic stewardess and this is what she has to say for herself:

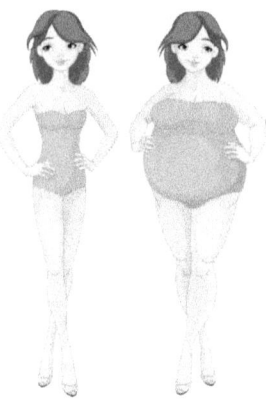

'Let me show you how I was two years ago. Look at this nice dress I was wearing at my sister's wedding. It looks purple here but its real colour is a really dark blue. I looked so fine in it. Look at my face, I had such defined cheekbones. Back then I could still wear short sleeves as my arms were still nice and slim. And my tummy, look at my tummy, it is so flat. These were the times when my ex boyfriend and I were going swimming twice a week, and running every other day of the week. These were the times when I spent so much time in the kitchen, cooking healthy food. These were the times when on Sundays I used to invite my girlfriends to have dinner and watch a movie together. These were the times when I'd wake up in the morning full of energy. These were the times when I didn't fly for a living!'

Penny   Which of these are you, Charlie?

Charlie   And you need to ask, darling? Surely the
               anorexic one! And you, Penny? Well, it's not
               so difficult to guess either. What do you think,
               Lilly? Who is she like?

Lilly   The nostalgic one maybe?

Charlie   Exactly so! And who will you become like,
               Lilly?

Lilly   For fuck's sake, none of them, I hope! I have
               another question for both of you. If you were to
               leave this job for good, what would be the
               aspect that you'd miss the most?

Penny   Buying cheap cigarettes abroad!

Charlie   C'mon Penny, be real! I'd say the human aspect
               of it which at the end for me is what really
               makes this job rewarding and precious.

Lilly   I certainly wasn't expecting that answer! The
               human aspect of your job is something I'm
               unfamiliar with. 'Tea or coffee sir?' and
               'Chicken or pork sir' is what people usually
               associate you with.

Charlie   Rescuing people at 35,000 ft. happens
               regularly, you just don't hear about it.
               Nevertheless, there's people who regularly
               faint; people who takes insulin but wrongly
               calculate the next time they are gong to eat,
               especially if the flight had been delayed;

people who are so scared to fly that they have very bad panic attacks; people who have epilepsy attacks; people whose eardrums blow up; people who die in their seats ... you name it, Lilly. However, there's a specific emergency situation we always hope that it will never happen: cardiac arrests. Although we have been trained for such emergencies, and retrained on it every 12 months, cardiac arrests are probably any hostess's worse nightmare. Likely, most of us have never had to experience it in their entire flying carrier, but unfortunately I don't belong in such a category. It did happen to me and I still remember it as if it had happened yesterday.

I was going somewhere in the States – I don't remember which city – and we were about an hour away from reaching our destination, when I saw my colleagues rescuing a man lying on the floor. I felt a sudden blast of fear. *I don't know what to do. What am I supposed to do? What equipment do I need? Where is the equipment I need? How do I use it? How do I put it together? If I don't know what I need, where it is, and how to use it, then I won't be able to do anything for this man's life. I am useless. I will never be able to forgive myself for the death of this man who is dying before my eyes. I have been trained to deal with these situations and now I can do nothing.*

And then, just when my own impeachment was about to turn nastier, and my questions uglier, someone nudged me on my shoulder and yelled at me: 'Grab the defibrillator! The man is unconscious. He's just had a heart attack!' The word 'defibrillator' then began to echo in my head. Its waves drowned my fears to death, and drench me to the skin with freezing water. I felt no fears any more, but felt no cold either. What I had become instead was pure power and energy, as if I had magically become a superwoman, equipped with magic tools, such as energy and power, which had now enabled me to think clearly and take action. I clearly saw the defibrillator in my head: it was inside a yellow container. I also saw where it was: in the dog-box by my jump seat. I then went for it. My legs were guiding me and my steps were taking me there. I opened the dog-box and sure enough the yellow container was just there. I grabbed it. I quickly joined the rest of my colleagues who were by the man. It was pure madness all around and everything was happening very quickly.

One of my colleagues was on top of the dying man and was giving him chest compressions. I heard her counting – '27, 28, 29, 30'. Then she stopped and my other colleague, who was opposite her, started giving the man two rescue breaths, mouth to mouth. I heard a loud 'Fuck' coming from my colleague's mouth, followed by 'He's vomiting! Someone grab me the aspirator at once!' The colleague standing next to me then took the aspirator, assembled it and threw it to my colleague, who plunged the long tube of the aspirator inside the man's throat and started to aspirate the vomit.

While doing so, the man was receiving more chest compressions from my colleague and I was putting the defibrillator together and getting ready to use it. Now the man's lips were blue and his skin was turning white. The man was not breathing any more and was unconscious: he was in cardiac arrest. I quickly wired him to the machine by placing two pads on his chest. My colleague stopped giving him chest compressions. I then turned the defibrillator on and followed the instructions in the defibrillator's display. It said that it was analysing the man's heart for any kind of activity, so I stood clear and waited for further instructions.

It then said that a shock was advised so I quickly cleared the immediate area from anyone or anything touching the man and I stood clear once again, ready to shock him as soon as the machine instructed me to do so. The machine said 'Clear to shock' so I pushed the green button. The man made a little jump from the ground, but nothing more, and the machine started to analyse his heart once again. While this was happening I was holding my breath in the hope that the machine would instruct me to shock him again, which would mean that there was still activity in his heart and that he could still be saved.

'No shock advised' the machine said. My eyes filled with tears, yet my grit grew even bigger. We started CPR on him once again, but this time it was another colleague of mine who was giving the man the chest compressions, as the previous one was now exhausted. The count started again '1, 2 , 3 ... 28, 29, 30. She stopped and my other colleague gave him two more rescue breaths mouth to mouth. Then the counting resumed again, followed by two rescue breaths. The man was still not breathing and was unconscious. We then prepared to shock him once again. As previously, I quickly wired the man to the machine, and my colleague stopped giving him chest compressions. I stood clear and waited for further instructions. The machine was analysing the man's heart. I held my breath once again. It said that a shock was advised and I was filled with joy and hope. I quickly cleared the immediate area from anyone and anything touching the man and stood clear, ready to shock him once again as soon as the machine instructed me to do so. The machine said 'Clear to shock' so I pushed the green button on the machine. The man made a little jump from the ground, and once again I held my breath for any vital signs. My colleague put his ear to the man's mouth to listen for his breaths. But the engines and air conditioning were loud. Unable to hear, he turned his head sideways and placed his cheek close to the man's mouth to feel the breaths instead. Meanwhile I, and all my colleagues, stood still, holding our breath, as if time had suddenly stopped.

'He's breathing,' he said.

We all exhaled in relief and inhaled the sound of such beautiful words. Although still unconscious, we immediately gave him some oxygen and placed him in the recovery position by pulling him onto his side. Two of us remained with the man to monitor him, while my other colleagues and I started to secure the cabin for immediate landing. As usual, we made sure passengers had their seatbelts fastened; that the aisles were clear of obstructions which might prevent people from quickly evacuating the plane in an emergency; and finally that passengers weren't wearing any kind of earphones, which might prevent them from hearing any sudden commands we might need to initiate in an emergency situation.

We then took our jump-seats by our respective doors and fastened ourselves as well. In front of me, just a few feet away, my two colleagues were monitoring the man, sitting on the floor just on top of the gear. I couldn't take my eyes away from them and kept repeating to myself, *Get this fucking plane on the ground safely! Don't smash the fucking tyres on the ground!* Then, on hearing the loud, incomparable sound of the gear coming down, my mind automatically switched into landing mode. All my senses were now on alert for anything unusual that might happen in or outside the cabin; I began to mentally run through the emergencies procedures, step by step; I envisioned myself in these procedures; I saw myself grabbing the fire extinguisher, torch, megaphone, opening the door, and shouting at passengers to quickly evacuate the plane; I recalled all the emergency announcements the pilots might make at any stage of landing and taxing, and how I was supposed to react to each and every one of them.

We were now just a few feet from the ground. I held my breath and waited for the tyres to touch the ground. We touched down smoothly. I immediately looked over at my colleagues sitting on the floor: they were fine. I saw one of them lowering his head towards the oxygen mask the man was wearing over his mouth and nose. He stared at it for a few seconds, waiting to see whether or not the mask held any sign of breathing. Then my colleague looked at me and put his thumb up. The man was alive and still breathing. Before I even realised it, the air bridge had been attached to my door, and I heard: 'Cabin crew, place doors to manual and cross-check.' I jumped off my seat and quickly opened the door. Paramedics rushed on board, placed the man on a stretcher and took him away at once. Soon after, the passengers disembarked. As they left, I stood by the door.

I clearly remember how hard it was to force a smile when passengers kept praising me as they walked by me, saying things like 'I can't believe you've saved that man's life' or 'I feel safer now to fly, knowing you are also trained to save people's lives' or 'That could have been *my* father.' However, they knew nothing of what I was going through at that moment as I forced a smile and waved them goodbye.

I was feeling extremely exhausted and feeble, as if I had just climbed a mountain, and felt drained of any emotions, as if my ability to feel anything, such as joy, accomplishment or even contentment, had been drawn off me. I felt detached from their praise, a victim of a terrible mistake that led these people to believe it was I who had saved this man's life, when in reality it was the superwoman I had magically once become but whose existence and even the smallest traces of her had now completely gone.

When all the passengers left, my colleagues and I sat down next to each other. Although we were all looking at each other, no one said a word to one another. We gave our statements of what had happened to the police and then quietly gathered our staff and left. On our way to the hotel, nobody talked on the bus either. Once we arrived at the hotel we were asked to change, take a shower, and meet downstairs in the hotel lounge in thirty minutes' time. The Captain then summoned us to sit down at a coffee table with a few beers on it.

'Grab a beer, guys,' the Captain said. We placed the beers between our legs, treasuring them, as if to lose sight of them meant we would have to look up and face the dreadful moment of looking each other in the eye. The Captain grabbed a beer as well and took a sip of it. He cleared his throat to get our attention, took a piece of paper out of his pocket and silently started to read it to recollect his thoughts and memorise what he was about to spell out. Next, he put the piece of paper back in his pocket and started to compliment us on the way we professionally and efficiently handled the medical emergency on board.

I clearly remember how the sound and meaning of such words, 'professionally' and 'efficiently', sparked a feeling of guilt and uneasiness in me; how these feelings of uneasiness and guilt turned me into a vulnerable human being.

If they only knew that it wasn't me who acted professionally and efficiently. If they only knew that the person sitting here didn't know what to do, or where the equipment was, or worse, how to use any equipment at all, they wouldn't say I had acted professionally and efficiently. On the contrary, they would think or maybe say I was an incompetent, unreliable person. I didn't do anything to save the man's life, they did. If it were down to me, that man would have died. I'm a liar because I'm deceiving people in believing it was me who saved his life when it wasn't me, but the superwoman I had become.

Then the guilt turned into pure shame and the thinking in my head ceased at once. All I wanted to do was to leave, hide, disappear. But the shame I was feeling had become so overwhelming that even the thought of making the slightest movement, such as simply blinking my eyes, became impossible. It was as if the shame had completely taken over my muscles, tied me to my chair, and prevented me from leaving. Luckily, a colleague of mine got up from his seat and excused himself for leaving. I quickly excused myself as well and tagged along after him . As we were about to enter the lift, the Captain stopped us.

'I called the hospital earlier and asked how the man was doing. You'll be glad to know that his granddaughter, who was waiting for him at the airport, had the chance to talk to him.'

I stood there in front of the Captain and said nothing. Yet I felt a sudden relief from the guilt I was carrying inside me, as images of the granddaughter kissing and talking to her grandpa kept flashing before my eyes, filling me with joy as I was looking at them.

'However,' the Captain continued, 'the hospital has just rang me to update me on the old man's status. Do you want to know if he's still alive?' the Captain asked us, and as he spoke those beautiful images in my mind abruptly metamorphosed into a horror movie.

In my mind now there is a movie screen. It projects the inside of a plane. The setting is familiar. It shows a man lying unconscious and not breathing on the floor and my colleagues trying to rescue him. However, although familiar, I'm nowhere to be seen in such a setting. I look closely at the frame in search of myself, but I'm not there. Then, when I am about to give up and resume watching the movie, I finally spot myself in the frame. I'm looking at my colleagues rescuing the man from afar, but I'm not helping them – I'm just looking at them. The man's face is out of focus, yet I can clearly make out his lips: they are blue. His body is also out of focus yet I can clearly make out his naked chest.

I look at his naked chest and stare at it. I inhale deeply, hold my breath in and wait for him to exhale. 'Fucking chest, move! Move!' I keep shouting to myself. And I keep staring at it and holding my breath in, yet he doesn't exhale – so I do it instead and then try one more time. I stare at his naked chest and inhale deeply, hold my breath in and wait for him to exhale – 'Move your damn chest, fucking move, move, move!' And I keep staring at it and holding my breath in, yet he doesn't exhale. So again I do it instead and exhale.

I start to shout at him at the top of my lungs! 'Move that fucking chest of yours! Fucking move it! Please move it!' But although I'm shouting, no sound is coming out of me, as if my vocal cords had been muted and the man can't hear me. I try to shout at the top of my lungs once again, but the same thing happens. I look at his face which I can now clearly see. His eyes are shut and his lips have turned purple. The skin has swollen and turned yellowish. Yet he looks serene.

'So, do you or don't you want to know if the man is still alive?' the Captain asks while nudging my shoulder to bring me back to reality.

'I don't want to know anything!' I yell at him and leave at once.

Lilly   Do you not know what happened to him?

Charlie   I never wanted to know, Lilly. I like to think he's happy and spending his remaining days with his granddaughter. And when he eventually dies, he will be surrounded by people who love and care for him.

Lilly   Were you able to take some time off? Did you ever get over it?

Charlie   We all came back to London as passengers because none of us had the mindset to work safely. Some of us took some time off, and some – me included – decided to go back to work as soon as possible. At first, the thought of operating and finding myself at 35,000 feet scared the hell out of me. I kept imagining walking through the cabin and finding a passenger lying on the floor, his lips purple, dying before my eyes.

I remember sitting on my jump seat and looking at the passengers just before take-off. I had spotted a few old, overweight passengers and thought to myself, 'Please don't have a heart attack!' I also remember how scared I was to walk through the cabin as I was scared at finding myself involved in yet another emergency situation. As time went on, my fears and guilt ceased to obsess me. What happened back then is now only a nightmare, but I keep asking myself if I'd react any differently if it were to happen ever again. I think I wouldn't, mainly because I've been trained to use a machine and follow procedures, not to deal with such extreme situations on a daily basis. Nurses and doctors are the ones who are constantly exposed to them all the time and grow accustomed to seeing purple lips and dead people, but we are not. So if it were to happen again, I would once again rely on my adrenaline to turn me into a superwoman and make me do what I learnt on manikins.

But if it were to happen again, I think I would cope with my emotions differently, because I realised that, although we are not nurses nor doctors, we can nevertheless do something rather than nothing at all. And that something is neither right nor wrong, it just is. So how can anyone feel guilty or shame when something has been done? I really need to go to the toilet now so Penny why don't you tell a story meanwhile?

Penny   Sure, a funny story! All this dying and rescuing business is making me sick to my stomach. I'll tell you a story about our super dry Crew Rest Area, the place where we rest for an hour or so in flight.

Lilly   Listen, Penny, I don't really care about your funny story and I don't give a damn about becoming a stewardess any more. And I don't wish to know why you girls are still doing this damn job either any more – and you know why? Because I know that everything you tell me would be pure bullshit.

Penny   What's got into you, Lilly? Have you gone mad?

Lilly   Never felt better, so let me talk. There has to be a very good reason to justify someone taking their own life and you have both made it clear to me tonight that this is exactly what this job is driving you to. However, what is more sick and disturbing is that although you're clearly aware of this, you and everybody else are still doing this job, despite knowing how bad it is for them.

Penny   I will turn my life around. I will put an end to it! I will!

Lilly   And that's very good but with all due respect, that's all to see in five years time, Penny. As for Charlie and all her stupid excuses, how can anyone with a bit of brain believe that it's OK to be lost and mindless when being lost and mindless is clearly turning her into a fucking walking zombie? You must confront her Penny! She needs serious help!

Penny   How can I confront someone who says how happy she is?

Lilly   Simple: you just do it! Bring up whatever happened that fateful night because it is whatever happened that night that is driving her to her own demise. You have told her that she is unhappy and miserable. Now tell her why! It's that simple! Just fucking do it! Not everything must have a reason in order to do it! You just fucking do it!

Penny   I don't have the guts, she's too aggressive, she scares me, she's too confident in herself.

Lilly   How will you feel then in five years' time when you turn your life around and she doesn't because you haven't had the guts to face her? Can you live with that?

Charlie   Am I interrupting anything?

Lilly   Actually—

Penny   Actually you are not! I was just about to tell Lilly the time when you scared the hell out of the passengers.

Charlie   What a scary moment that was!

Lilly   Actually I'm quite tired, ladies, and I'm going back to the hotel if you don't mind.

Charlie   We'll tag along then, it's getting quite late for us too.

Lilly   If you don't mind, Charlie, I prefer to have some time with myself. Also I have decided to stay in Rome a day longer. So I won't come back with you tomorrow.

Charlie   As you wish, Lilly, but are you OK?

Lilly   Actually I'm not OK, Charlie!

Charlie   Is there anything we can do to help you?

Lilly   You have already! In fact, I want to take this opportunity to thank you both very much for having shone some light on what I mistakenly and naively thought to be the most perfect and enviable job on earth. Although you have stripped me of my dream, I am still truly grateful to have had the chance to meet you and know you as people, rather than as air stewardesses.

Charlie   It could be a fun job, and certainly is for those air stewardesses who still live at home with their parents, or have a partner who has a 'real' job and can effort to work part time—

Penny   Ergo flying becomes more a hobby rather than a job, you mean!

Lilly   I wish! But for now I'm looking more for a career path than a hobby to occupy my time! Have a good night, and thank you again for everything.

Charlie   Lilly, wait! Is there anything you have forgotten to ask us?

Lilly   Not really, is there?

Charlie   The question you've kept asking us all night: why in hell we are still doing this job?

Lilly   Actually, Charlie, I didn't forget. I would rather ask you that question in five years' time when we will all three meet at this very restaurant and you can tell me more stories about the time you used to fly!

Penny   It sounds good, Lilly! Good night and see you in five years!

Charlie   See you in five years, Lilly!

Lilly   Take care of yourselves!

*

As I'm leaving them behind, I can't help feeling a sense of sadness crawling on me, so I decide to walk back to the hotel rather than take a taxi. I don't really know where I'm going, but I keep walking where my legs are taking me. It's past midnight and most of the restaurants and pubs are shut already. The streets are dark and deserted, apart from a few dogs walking about and couples kissing.

I venture through a few alleys and cross a few bridges, until I stumble on the Trevi Fountain. It is all illuminated and it looks even more magical and theatrical than earlier. I can't take my eyes off of it. I'm hypnotised by its beauty!

I catch my breath and carry on walking. As I come closer to the fountain, it looks as if the statues are moving and talking to me: horses and their riders seem to dance and in doing so, they welcome me to do the same. So I do. I stretch my arms up high in the sky and I let my body be guided by a sudden sense of freedom. Before I know it I'm dancing, spinning and twirling as if I had magically become a ballerina performing on stage.

As I go closer to the fountain, I catch a glimpse of some sparks. I stop dancing and walk towards the fountain. The sparks increase as I approach. 'They are coming from the water!' I say aloud. 'The water is sparkling with thousands of different little lights!' I look down into the water and the bottom is covered with coins.

I immerse my left arm into the water and take a bunch of coins in my hand. When I open my hand, the world opens up before my eyes: each coin comes from a different part of the world. No one coin is alike! *Thousand of people around the world*, I think, *have come here and tossed a coin into the water in the hope of fulfilling their dreams, just as I have. How many of these dreams have been broken and faded like mine?*

I put the coins back into the water with all the other thousands of coins sitting at the bottom and I walk around the edge of the fountain. I stop where I had thrown my coin from earlier and look down at the bottom so as to see what a broken dream looks like. I see no broken dreams anywhere, let alone mine! *Where has it gone? Where have all the broken dreams gone?* I walk along the edge of the fountain, but I see only sparkling coins, dancing, spinning and twirling as if they were ballerinas.

The phrase SEE THE WORLD BETTER jumps in my mind yet again and I magically see the world with the eyes of dreams. 'No broken dream exists because dreams only exist if one truly believes in them, and sparkle and dance only when nurtured and cared for!' I say aloud. 'My dream of becoming an air hostess has never been nothing more than an infatuation, which was born in Barbados and later faded with Penny and Charlie's accounts of flying. How can I ever find it in here then?'

I reach inside my pocket and take a coin. Before I toss it into the water, I think of something I can truly believe in and nurture: I visualise my dream of becoming a successful psychologist, and then I throw the coin. As I hear my coin touching the bottom of the fountain, I feel a sense of relief, as if a heavy burden of fears and doubts had just been lifted from my shoulder: I now feel lighter, stronger, invincible!

I run towards a main road and grab a cab back to the hotel. I'm very excited and can't wait to tell Penny about the magical fountain, the dancing statues, sparkling water, and thousands of ballerinas. I quickly pay the taxi driver and run to the room but to my disappointment Penny is already asleep.

I put my pijamas on and go under the blankets next to Penny. Before I secure my sleeping position, I whisper her name. She doesn't say anything, yet she acknowledges me by murmuring something I don't understand.

'Penny, you must see the world with the eyes of dreams!' I tell her.

'Really Lilly? And how on earth am I to do that?'

'You must visit the Trevi Fountain by night! And Charlie too! It's magical! Just go there!'

'That's great, Lilly! But what good can it be to go there when I don't believe in freaking dreams in the first place?'

'Penny, I kid you not! Thousands of dreams are dancing, spinning and twirling in the water! It's magical! Dreams are magical! They turn you into a ballerina. They make you free and invincible.'

'It's late, Lilly. Go to sleep. We'll talk again tomorrow.'

I turn around and a little while later I fall asleep. When I wake up in the morning, Penny has already left.

FOUR   FIVE YEARS LATER

'Flight 2222 to Rome. Last call for Lilly Smith.'

I hear the announcement loud and clear, but I can't run any faster. When I finally arrive at my gate I'm out of breath and can't speak. I hand my boarding pass and passport to the stewardess behind the desk and keep running down the jetty towards the aircraft. I show my boarding pass once again to the stewardess standing by the door. As soon as I step inside the plane, the stewardess closes the door behind me.

'I'm very thirsty. Can I please have a glass of water?' I ask the stewardess as I desperately try to catch my breath.

'We will come around with beverages shortly after take-off. Now please go to your seat, madam,' she tells me. I want to insist but I daren't say another word after such a clear and sharp response, so I obey and go and sit down.

After ten minutes, which seems like an eternity, the plane moves and shortly after we take off. I wait for the seatbelt sign to go off and as soon as it does I push the call bell. I wait for a stewardess to come over but nobody does. My throat is now very dry and I struggle to swallow. I decide to go and get it myself but it's not as easy as it might sound, I'm afraid: I am sitting by the window and the two passengers sitting next to me are fast asleep.

It's surely cruel of me to wake them up, I think, *but I have no choice: I need to drink some water now.*

Luckily, just as I'm about to wake them up, I see a stewardess walking down the aisle. Relieved, I look at her to grab her attention, but she doesn't seem to acknowledge my effort.

It's OK, I think, *surely she can't miss the big red light shining above my head.* She's getting ever closer to me, yet she pays no attention to me and sure enough walks past me.

Damn you woman! You shamelessly avoided me! OK then, I'll go and get it myself!

I touch the shoulder of the person sitting next to me, but he doesn't wake up. I try again and this time I apply a bit more pressure when I do it. Nothing, he doesn't move.

I swear this is the last time I will ever sit next to the damn window! I think while looking at both the men who are blocking me. *There's no way I can walk by them without sitting on their crotches for crying out loud! I have to wake them up! I have to get out of here.*

I gently shake both of them one by one several times but neither of them wakes up.

Great! And now? How do I fucking get out of here!

I look out of the window in total despair but all I can see before my eyes is my rage marching in. I start to cough uncontrollably and while I'm doing it I nudge the person sitting next to me. I stop and look over them but both of them are impassive and unresponsive to my strategy to wake them up.

For crying out loud! How can anyone sleep in a plane, let alone so damn deeply? I push the call bell several times and then look around to see if anyone would appear. No sign of them.

I've had it! I think and stand up but as I'm doing it I catch sight of two stewardess talking in front of the plane. One of them is coming towards me so I happily sit back down. I flap my hand in the air but she keeps ignoring me. I wave both my hands then frenetically, yet the inevitable happens: she walks past me! Bewildered for the first second but enraged for the next I shout at the top of my lungs: 'Excuse me miss!'

She comes to a sudden and complete stop, turns her body around in slow emotion, and marches towards me. When she gets to me, she looks right at me and says, 'Is there a problem, madam?'

'Well, I would like a glass of water please.'

'A glass of water?' She asks in a patronising manner. Then, just as condescendingly, she continues: 'Madam, let me tell you something: the call bell is to be used only for emergencies. Surely, a glass of water is not an emergency, is it now?'

'Surely,' I reply, 'it's not and I can ensure you that if it weren't for these two people who are blocking me, I wouldn't—'

She walks away while I'm still speaking.

That's it, now you've really made my blood boil, stewardess Ruth!

I get up and start trying to climb over the man sitting next to me but he's too big and I give up. I sit back down again and try to calm myself down. *How pointless it would be to confront anyone who can wake up every morning and go on doing something that she absolutely hates and despises!* I think. I find a sense of relief in those words, but then Charlie and Penny come into my mind and I get goosebumps.

What if they have turned just as miserable as this stewardess? No way! They will both be at the restaurant looking fabulous and healthier than me! I look behind me and two stewardesses are pushing a trolley down the aisle. I count four rows ahead of me. I wait my turn patiently.

What if Charlie is still flying? No fucking way, Penny would have never allowed it to happen.

'Madam, would you like anything to drink?'

'Sure Ruth! I would like ten glasses of water, thank you.'

'I can give you only two, madam.'

'Then I want a bottle of water, *madam*.'

She gives me the bottle of water without saying a word. I happily take it! And she moves on.

I drink my water and I close my eyes in sight of great relief. Shortly after I close my eyes and rest.

Half hour before landing, the passengers sitting next to me finally wake up. I smile in relief. I take my toilet bag and happily ask them to get up and let me through. Both toilets in the back of the aircraft are occupied so I wait by the galley where both of the stewardesses are, including Ruth.

They are sitting on their jump seats and eating. I can't help noticing the amount of food on top of the counter. I look at it in disbelief: there's one plate with what looks like beef floating in heavy brown sauce; another has what looks like chicken swimming in a heavy yellow sauce; another has rigatoni pasta in heavy white sauce; another has desserts – one looks like a chocolate mousse, the other cheesecake. Also on their laps are two more plates: one is eating gnocchi in white sauce and the other's eating bread and cheese.

When they notice me standing there, I leave and go to the toilet. I wash my face in cold water, brush my teeth and put some make-up on. I then go to the galley again. All the plates on the counter are empty; they have eaten them all and are now eating the desserts. *No doubt they both belong to the 'Neurotic' category of stewardesses!* I smile to myself.

'Sorry to interrupt your lunch, ladies, but is there any chance I can have a cup of coffee from you?' I ask.

Ruth doesn't even acknowledge my question, but luckily Betty does. She stands up and starts to brew some fresh coffee. While I'm waiting, I make conversation with Betty.

'How long have you been doing this job?' I ask her.

'Three years now.'

'Are you planning to do it for the rest of your life?'

'Not really. One more year and then I'll do something else.'

'Do you already know what you will do?'

'I haven't really decided yet, but I will. Surely I will!' She gives me my coffee and resumes talking: 'I saw this film a few weeks ago where this guy had a big banner hanging on his bedroom wall. The banner was made out of five pieces of square cardboard and each cardboard had a letter. The phrase read: I WILL. I thought what a great motivational phrase. So I went to Ikea and bought the magic five letters so I could also hang them on my bedroom wall. But I never did so! Oh well...'

I'm standing there, waiting for her to add something more to her story but she doesn't. She pours a cup of coffee for herself instead, starts to drink it and while looking at me she asks, 'Do you need anything else?' I want to ask her if she sees any paradox in what she has just said, but I bite my tongue and I excuse myself instead.

I'm back to my seat and I take out the red envelope with my name on it. Ever since I had it, I have been keeping it inside the little pockets of my handbags.

Despite what they might have decided to do of their lives, I think, *it'll be nice to catch up with them after such long time. But that's a lie and you know it! You would be extremely disappointed if they are indeed still flying. Our friendship would surely take a turn for the worse. After all what could I possibly do, or say for that matter, after they have chosen to cut their brains into pieces and hand them out to the airline to devour? Now calm down, you are just getting too anxious. We will all three sit down and tell each other about our successful lives and great achievements! Stop worrying!*

The stewardesses are securing the cabin. We are landing. 'Miss, fasten your seat belt please,' Betty tells me. I look at her eyes and they remind me of Charlie's: they are sad. I look at her skin and it reminds me of Penny's: it is dry and yellowish. *What excuses have you built for yourself to destroy your hopes and dreams? Is it the lack of alternatives? Or is it the joy of being mindless?*

'Madam, will you please fasten your seatbelt?'

Why don't you come with me and meet Charlie and Penny? So you can see with your own eyes that it is indeed possible to change your miserable life.

'Madam, please fasten your seatbelt.'

Woman, you look so tired. Ten hours of sleep right now wouldn't do you any good, but thirty-six hours would surely help you.

'Madam, fasten your seatbelt!'

How many caffeine pills have you taken today to stay awake?

'Is there a problem, madam, are you OK?' Betty asks while shaking me.

'A problem? Not really. Why?'

'I've asked you to fasten your seat belt four times!'

'Sorry! I was lost in my own thoughts'.

We land in Rome and once outside the airport I go and fetch a taxi. I tell the taxi driver to take me straight to the restaurant. The traffic is just as bad as I remembered it. By the time I finally arrive to the restaurant, I'm thirty minutes late. I gaze through each table outside the place, but I can't see either of them. I sit down at one table and when the waiter comes I order a bottle of red wine and three glasses, and I wait.

Thirty minutes go by but still no sign of either of them. I walk inside the restaurant and ask if anyone has maybe called and asked for me. Nobody has. So I go back to my table and keep waiting and looking around. After having waited for nearly two hours, I begin to accept that they will never show up. I picture them still working at 35,000 feet and my heart fills with tears and rage. I take the red envelope out of my handbag and open it. The paper only reads: *I can do it. I must do it. I will do it.* I take my lighter and am about to set the paper alight when I see someone running from afar. As she comes closer I can make out her features: it's Penny! I stand up and start waving to her.

'I'm here!' I shout.

She sees me and comes towards me.

'Sorry I'm late,' she says, hugging me. Then she releases me and looks around frantically. 'Where is Charlie? Lilly, where is Charlie?'

'Calm down, Penny. She's not here yet. She must be late too.'

'She won't come, Lilly, and it's all my fault.'

'Have a glass of water and sit down. We can call her and see where she is. Give me her phone number, I'll call her.'

'You don't understand, Lilly, she won't come.'

'Stop worrying. Give me her phone number.'

'I don't have it any more.'

The word 'any more' starts echoing in my mind.

'What do you mean *any more,* Penny? What happened between you two?'

'That night, when you left us at the restaurant, I tried to talk to her but she lost it as soon as I asked her to tell me what happened the night she stood me up for lunch. She got up and left me there without saying a word to me. A few days later I called her but she had changed her phone number already. I went to her house several times, but she never answered and let me in. I saw her a few times at work. At first she completely avoided me, despite my attempts to talk to her. Then one time she took me on the side and told me to go away and to leave her alone. So I did.'

'Nevertheless, have you seeing her at work or received news of her?'

'I left the airline about two years ago and she was still there. I haven't heard or seen her since.'

'OK, let's both calm down. She might just be late so let's wait. Now, tell me about you. You look so different, I almost didn't recognise you! Your hair is so long now! You look fabulous! And I love your dress! Tell me, I want to know everything! What do you do now?'

'I'm a health and beauty practitioner. Shortly after our conversation in Rome, I applied to work part-time and went back to school. When I received my diploma three years later, I quit flying and found a job in a beauty salon in London. It wasn't at all easy at first, but now I'm so happy and regret not having done it much earlier!'

'That's great, Penny. You have turned your life around! You did it!'

'There's more, Lilly. My grandma has recently died and left me a bit of money. I want to use it to open my own health and beauty practice with Charlie. I want Charlie to be part of it too. I've been waiting for this day so impatiently to tell her this.'

'Listen, you will, and even if she won't show up today, we will track her down, wherever she is the world, and you will tell her. So what I propose to do now is to toast to your success.'

I raise my glass but Penny doesn't. Instead she looks surprised and scared as if she has just seen a ghost appearing behind my shoulders. I quickly turn around to look and then I see her, standing behind me.

'Sally, what are you doing here?' Penny asks inquisitively yet concerned.

'You were expecting to see Charlie, weren't you?' Sally asks.

'Yes we were, but why are you here, Sally?' I ask.

'Where is Charlie, Sally? Did she tell you to come on her behalf?' Penny asks.

'Then you don't know, do you?' Sally says with a concerned tone.

'What is it that we don't know, Sally? Has something happened to Charlie?' Penny dares to ask.

Sally takes a chair from a nearby table and carries it over to Penny and Lilly's table, then she lights up a cigarette for herself, sits down and begins to give her account of Charlie's past few years.

'About two years ago Charlie came to visit me and asked if she could stay at my place for free until she had enough money to start paying for rent. Since I was planning to live abroad for a few months and I was looking for someone to look after my cats, I invited her to move in as soon as she could without questioning her. So she did and shortly after I left for France.

'When I came back home six months later and she came at the door I couldn't recognise her: she looked ill, exhausted and terribly sad. Of course I asked her immediately what the matter was and though she said it was nice of me to show interest in her well-being, there was nothing to worry about because she had already gone to see a doctor, performed a series of tests, and excluded all major diseases. But when I asked her again to tell me why she had lost so much weight if it wasn't for some serious illness, she was reluctant to answer me and instead asked me about my time in France. As you can imagine alarms bells started to ring immediately because it was obvious that there had to be more to her story that met the eye. I kept pressing her to explain why she had become so thin, but she kept changing the subject and finally left to go to work.

'But that same afternoon I happened to stumble upon her roster, which she had left in the toilet accidentally that morning before going to work, and learned that she had gone back working full time. It was right then that I understood why she had fallen ill, for I had seen it happening way too many times to my fellow colleagues and even experienced it myself when I was still flying.'

Penny quickly jumps in and adds, 'The massive workload, back-to-back long-haul trips and jetlag, coupled with not having had enough days off to recuperate or catch up with sleep, caused her health to deteriorate.'

'Exactly,' Sally says, then taking a drag of her cigarette resumes talking. 'Yet, I couldn't understand why in hell she had decided not to tell me about having gone back to work full time, or worse why she had gone back working full time in the first place, so I asked her just that as soon as we sat down for dinner later that evening when she came back from work.

'She calmly confessed that eventually she would have told me about it, and that she hadn't because I had already left for France when she had gone back working full time. Although I could have easily argued that on the contrary she had plenty of chances to tell me about it when we had spoken on the phone while I was in France, I didn't. Instead, I asked her why she had decided to work full time knowing exactly how badly it had affected her health in the past. She replied that she had no choice because she had drained all her savings and couldn't rely on the little money she was earning working part time any more. In other words, she was skint, so she had no other choice than going back to work full time.

'Although it might have been a plausible reason for most people, nonetheless such an answer caught me off guard, as you can imagine, for the Charlie I knew and had known for some time would never have said that there were no choices. In fact, one of her strongest beliefs was that every problem always has a solution for there are many choices we can make to resolve it. I still thought that maybe I could have misunderstood her or that she hadn't expressed herself properly, so I calmly replied as she would have done if she were in my shoes in the hope of awakening some sense on her. I told her that by all means she had many choices, for she could have opted to go back into what she used to do before starting to fly, for instance, instead of going back working full time.'

'For crying out loud, Sally! Stop talking as if you were writing an essay for some damn university! Cut to the chase! Just tell us what happened to Charlie! *Pleeease!*'

'Let her fucking talk, Lilly! Don't interrupt her, damn it! I want to know what Charlie had to say for herself,' says Penny. 'Besides,' she says to me, 'this is how she normally talks, so sit tight or else we could be still sitting here tomorrow!'

'Well, Penny', Sally sighs, 'she said nothing about it! She simply went ballistic on me! She stood up in front of me, and while pointing her finger at me, told me at the top of her lungs that it wasn't any of my business to interfere with her decision and that I was never again to speak about what she used to do because it was history and she would never go back to being a lawyer nor doing anything else related to law.

'Needless to say, such an abrupt, inappropriate reaction raised even more alarm bells in my head, for it could only have come out if she had a serious issue with her past and with being a lawyer. If this was the case, I thought, then most likely she was still flying because she felt trapped in her job.'

On hearing these words, Penny seizes Sally by her arm. 'Did you ask her why she didn't want to be a lawyer any more? Did she tell you why she didn't want to talk about her past or what happened back then?'

'OK that's enough you two!' says Sally. 'You have to stop getting in my hair all the time! I understand you are both anxious to know what happened to Charlie, but it's crucial you know why. So please let me talk and be patient.'

'Then something did happen to Charlie! Something bad!' Penny says, covering her face with both hands in quiet desperation. So I quickly take Penny in my arms and after having soothed her with assuring words, I sign Sally to go on, which she does without any apparent objection.

'Since she was quite upset I couldn't ask her any questions, Penny. After I calmed her down and assured her that my intentions were benevolent, I kept pressing her to explain about her choice to keep flying in the hope of encouraging her to confide in me whatever it was that was preventing her from quitting flying. I asked her how much longer she planned to work full time. She started to act as if she had lost her marbles. But just when I was about to repeat the question, she started telling me how much she loved her job because it gave her the chance to help other people.'

'What? Loved her job because it gave her the chance to help other people?' Penny says in disbelief.

'Has she gone totally mad?' we both said.

'Why then,' I add, 'didn't she choose to become a nurse instead, or God knows what, if she loved helping people so much? Being a nurse could have rewarded her just as much, without ruining her health!'

'That's exactly what I thought too when I heard such blasphemous words coming from her mouth! I honestly couldn't believe my ears and my facial expression must have given it away because in her pitiful attempt to convince me otherwise, she kept going on and on about how flying had given her many opportunities to help people. Don't get me wrong – all her stories were quite amusing and captivating. In one, for instance, she saved someone's life who had suffered from an heart attack, but that's all they were, because they completely failed to persuade me to change my mind. In fact, if anything at all, they confirmed what I had dared to think ever since she had gone ballistic on me—'

'That her past must have got the better of her,' Penny jumps in, 'and she must have given way to a miserable life, just as my lack of self-confidence succeeded in frightening me away from moving on in life for a long time.'

'Exactly,' says Sally. 'Fear is like a plague: a highly contagious disease that grows and rapidly spreads in people's minds. It spares no one, not even the strongest or most confident person like Charlie. Some people try to cover up their worst fears by pretending to be happy, just as Charlie was doing, or by claiming to be unhappy, just as you did, Penny, or by ignoring it all together, just as I did with mine. But fear is neither a fool nor a gullible feeling. It will constantly confront us and challenge our minds until it achieves what it was set on doing from the very beginning: driving our lives to destruction.

'Just think for a moment of all the people you know who are indeed clearly unhappy or on the contrary apparently happy but secretly miserable. The world is full of them and they can be found all over – at work, on the streets, in the underground, and even living with you. The ones who declare they are unhappy might complain, wish for a better life and criticise whoever is better off and more content than them, while the self-deceiving ones may pretend to be happy, boast about being content, and challenge whoever questions their happiness. But ultimately they are all equally resentful about their lives and the way they have turned out, regardless of what they pretend or not to be.

'Yet they do nothing to change their lives. On the contrary they hold on to the very thing that is causing them such bitter, sorrowful existence, like a disrespectful husband is for someone or an underpaid job might be for somebody else. Even so, deep inside they all secretly long to break away one day from their miserable relationships and start a new life, or find a job that betters their qualifications and rewards their skills. Yet they manage to bury their dreams six feet under and live their nightmares instead.'

'Just as Charlie has buried her dream of being a lawyer ever again and lived her nightmare of flying for the rest of her life,' Penny adds.

'Indeed, Penny. Have you ever wondered why these people are so loath to turn their lives around? I have, when at one point in my life I finally found the courage to come to terms with the very choices I alone had made over the years, that had caused my life to turn into a living hell and for me to ultimately loathe myself.

'You see, ever since I was a teenager I dreamed of having my own florist shop, yet I never dared tell anyone about this because I feared what people might think of me if I told them I wanted to sell flowers for a living. I was terribly ashamed of it. So instead of following my dream I kept it strategically hidden from anyone by choosing a career that people worship – and became part of a glamorous cabin crew. Although I loved it at first, when I started to see what it was doing to my health and realised that it wouldn't have taken me anywhere career wise, I began to panic.

'I knew right there and then that the best thing to do was to look for another job. Yet in my mind there was only one other possible job: the job I was ashamed of. So I talked myself into believing I had no other choice than to hang on to flying by telling myself a few white lies that lured me into thinking there wasn't any other career apart from flying that would have just as equally concealed my shame in selling flowers for a living. Little did I know back then that in doing so I had just started to lay the ground for more and bigger lies to come my way every time I needed to justify my choice of hanging on to flying. Moreover, all these lies would ultimate jeopardise my happiness and eventually bring me down a peg.

'One of the most infamous lies I used to keep holding on to my job, was when I told myself it was OK to have backache on a daily basis, or to be constantly deprived of sleep, or perpetually lack energy to do anything, because everybody with whom I worked had the same symptoms and were just as exhausted as I. Therefore, I not only grew accustomed to being in pain all the time, but I also made myself believe that I didn't need to find another job anymore.

'However, it wasn't until I reached the lowest point in my life that I finally realised how my own lies had contributed the building of my fabricated life in which I was able to manipulate reality to endorse my choice to hang on to my job. Furthermore, my lies had formed the foundation of what later turned into a point of no return. In fact, since my life had become the sum of all my lies, over time I grew so obliged to them with the commitment to tell more lies, that changing my life around became, or so I strongly believed, virtually impossible to accomplish because it implied that I had to undo all the lies I had been telling myself and people around me for years.'

'I can't follow all your words any longer, Sally,' Penny says. 'I apologise if I'm being abrupt but Lilly and I came here to meet Charlie, and she isn't here and we find you instead who happens to know something about Charlie. We've been here for more than an hour and we still don't fucking know what's happened to her. Now, although your story is very interesting, with all due respect, this is neither the time nor place to tell us about you.'

Penny and I stare at Sally waiting for a reply, and although she remains silent, her frozen body speaks on her behalf. After a few seconds she starts talking as if nothing has just happened.

'As you wish then! Cutting a long story short, one day in despair I drew a line in the sand. I gave my notice in to my manager, returned my uniform to the airline and asked my mother to loan me some money. Then without looking back or knowing exactly where, what and how I would have gone about it, I packed my suitcase with a few clothes and went to France to follow my dream. When I came back home six months later, I had a successful florist shop running in a small town in France.'

'Was it this the time you also saw Charlie?' I ask.

'Yes it was. So when I realised that Charlie was living a fabricated life and was just as trapped and hopeless as I had been before I left for France, I thought that the best way to rescue her was by merely supporting her. I wanted to show her that it was still possible to have her life even if she had betrayed her dreams. After all people are much better at taking somebody else's advice rather than their own, and Charlie is surely no exception! So I told her how miserable my life was before I decided to move to France and how I had overcome my fears and ultimately followed my dream.

'After carefully listening to me, she hugged me and broke into uncontrollable tears. I let her cry and when she calmed down she relieved her mind and heart of all the fears that ultimately had taken over her life. She said that flying had become her way to punish herself for having caused the death of a man. And that she was totally aware of the fact that flying was taking her six feet under. But this was precisely what she wanted because she thought she deserved to be miserable.'

'Wait a second, Sally! What are you saying? That she killed someone?' I mumble.

'Well, that was what she thought. She told me that one day she received a phone call from the mother of a man she had sent to prison when she was still a lawyer in France. Apparently this man had taken his life and the mother accused Charlie of her son's death.'

'How can it be when Charlie had merely done her job: sending a guilty man to prison?' I say and Penny adds, 'And how she could have killed him if he was in prison?'

'Well, this man had another trial that had proven him innocent of all those crimes that Charlie had initially sent him to jail for. So after having spent some time in prison he was set free and shortly after he killed himself.'

'And the mother blamed Charlie for having caused the pain that ultimately drove her son to suicide. Is that it?' I say.

'Not exactly. Before he hung himself her son wrote a letter to explain all the reasons that had brought him to take his life. He said that his life, ever since he had being accused of murdering his neighbour, had become a living hell because although he had later been proven innocent, people were still treating him as a criminal and a murderer. If her lawyer had done her job properly in the first place, he wrote, people would have never placed the stigma on him that ruined his life and ultimately caused him to take his own life.'

'Now everything is clear', Penny says. 'This must have happened the night she showed up at my place after having disappeared all day long. She told me she was over with the law and with being a lawyer. Receiving this phone call couldn't have happened at a worse time in her life as I now recall the conversation we had just a few days earlier at the park, when Charlie had told me how each unsuccessful interview was bringing her down and taking a toll on her self esteem. Poor Charlie, it must have been horrible to live with such guilt and not be able to talk about it.'

'That's exactly what she had told me and after I helped her reason through the ordeal and convinced her that she had done nothing wrong but her job, and that she wasn't responsible for this man's life, I encouraged her to start her life all over again by putting her past where it belonged once and for all. So I invited her to come to France with me and become my business partner and help run my florist shop. She didn't hesitate to accept my invitation. In fact, she was so enthusiastic and happy that she couldn't even breathe! I had never seen her so happy, as if a big burden had just been released from her mind, soul and body!'

'And it took you an hour to tell us that Charlie is happily living in France?' Penny asks disappointed.

'Why didn't you tell us right from the very beginning that she was in France?' I ask.

Sally ignores us. 'We started making plans that same night. We decided she would give her resignation from work as soon as she came back from Orlando in three days' time, and that we would leave in three weeks' time. We bought the tickets to go to France that night! She asked me to show her the pictures of the town that was soon to become her home; and the pictures of my florist shop; and the picture of my place in France and—'

'You are doing it again, Sally,' Penny interrupts but Sally shushes her. 'Since she looked particularly tired, just before she was going to bed, I asked her if she wanted to borrow my car to go to work the following day instead of taking the train so she could sleep another hour in the morning. She happily accepted my offer.

Three days later she calls me from the airport to tell me that her flight had just landed with an hour's delay and that she would be home by eleven at the latest. However, at two o'clock she still wasn't home. Although concerned, I wasn't worried because I thought that she might have parked somewhere en route to take a power nap in the car. After all, we all know how exhausted one can be after having come back from long haul and having worked all night long. However, about an hour later, I receive a phone call from a police officer who told me that my car had been involved in a car crash and that a woman by the name of Charlie Dover was driving my car.'

Both Penny and I gasped – and neither of us said a word.

'When I told her that I knew her, the officer told me to rush to the hospital right away, so I called a taxi. On my way there I kept blaming myself for whatever might have happened to Charlie. Mainly because I should have taken her to the airport. I shouldn't have allowed her to drive my car. I should have given her a ride to the airport and picked her up when she returned from Orlando. How would she know how dangerous and imprudent it is to drive home right after coming back from work? She always took a train. I should have known better, I should have driven her to work, damn it!

'When I arrived, the officer told me exactly what I was fearing the most – that Charlie had fallen asleep at the wheel and hit a tree. The impact had been so violent that she had been thrown out of the car and landed a few yards away from the car. When they found her, although motionless, she was still alive, and she was rushed to the nearest hospital.'

'And …?' Penny asked.

'She's in my house. I've been taking care of her for the past two years.'

'Taking care of?' – I mumble – 'What does that mean?'

Sally hesitates and then looks both Penny and me in the eye. 'She's been in a coma and relying on life-support machines ever since her car crash.'

*

The world around me becomes distant and surreal, as if I have suddenly become a spectator rather than its inhabitant. I see people moving in slow emotion. They scream but I can't hear them. They run but they don't advance. I turn my head to one side and I see a disfigured face depicting fear. I look at it and I recognise the face: it's Penny's. Her mouth is wide open and she's uttering something but I can't hear what she's shouting. The world around me starts to pick up some pace and without any warning I hear a loud 'No' coming from Penny's mouth and she blacks out.

Shortly after, the paramedics come. They bring her back and place her on a stretcher. Once inside the ambulance they put an oxygen mask over her mouth and nose and attach a few wires on her chest.

'If you wish to speak to her now, you can,' the paramedic says while moving away from Penny and indicating to us to sit by her, which we do.

We both get hold of Penny's hands. Although none of us is talking, nevertheless we all find plenty of thoughts and feelings to share and pain to soothe. Only when we arrive at the hospital do we let go of our hands.

After a few hours we leave the hospital. Sally asks me where the taxi should take us. I tell her the Hilton Hotel. When the taxi arrives Penny and I hug Sally and get inside the taxi. Sally is waving goodbye from the side walk. Then just when the taxi has moved, Penny tells the taxi driver to stop. She rolls down the window and asks Sally to come closer.

'How did you know about our meeting?' she asks her.

Sally reaches inside her handbag and hands her a clear plastic bag. Inside, there were lots of heart stickers and a red envelope. 'It was in Charlie's handbag when she had the accident,' Sally says.

They look at each other without saying a word then Penny signals to the driver to leave.

Penny is holding the plastic bag in her hands.

'I let her down, Lilly! If only I had the guts to stand up to her and tell her to vomit whatever it was that was poisoning her existence and subverting the course of her life, this wouldn't have happened. If I am where I am today, I owe it solely to her. She was the one who encouraged me to face my hypocrisy and deal with my stupid insecurity. She was the one who gave me the strength to change my life around. And what have I done in return for her? Nothing but let her swim in her own pile of shit! While I was building a life for myself.'

'Listen, Penny, I'm just as guilty as you are. If I had tried harder to encourage you into talking with her that night in Rome, you most likely would have done it. Besides, I could have just as well been the one who stood up to her, but I didn't and went on building my life. After all you told me what had happened to her that fateful night!

'So many useless *ifs!* The truth is that I have failed in giving her support! So now what? How good can my life ever be when the very person who had made it all possible, is not in it?'

For the rest of our journey neither of us dared to say one more word. We didn't leave our respective bedrooms for days, until one day Sally came to our rescue and told us about her plan to write a memoir.

FIVE   ONE YEAR LATER

THE BEGINNING OF
THE END

Just as I park in front of Penny's place she comes out of her building with two big suitcases. I shout from the car to ask if she needs any help carrying them but she doesn't reply nor acknowledge my question. I dare not ask her again – or say anything for that matter – because I know that she is furious with me and that she's just waiting to get in my car to start lecturing me. So I diligently wait for her inside the car.

'Lilly, you are late, again! You were supposed to be here at six o'clock and it's now half past six! ... But this time you'll call Sally and you'll tell her that we are running late.'

'I can't do it, I'm driving.'

'This excuse has served you well for too many times, but it won't today, missy! I've got you some useful earphones that I'm now going to plug into your phone so that you can call her while driving. Now put them on and I'll dial Sally's number for you.'

'It's not safe to drive with this things in my ears. I can't drive and talk on the phone, Penny. I need to focus, to concentrate! C'mon, Penny, just do it! You could have done it already if you hadn't wasted all this time complaining about it.'

'Fine then, I will do it, but I swear that this will be the last time! Last time, Lilly! Did you hear me!'

Penny dials Sally's phone number and only after one ring Sally picks up the phone.

'If you're calling to tell me that you are late yet again, you better have a good excuse,' Sally says with a calm yet angry tone. Then she pauses for a few seconds to give Penny the chance to speak but as soon as Penny mumbles the word 'well', Sally shushes her and goes ballistic on her.

'I really don't give a damn, excuse my French, to know why you are late because it won't change the situation. I have begged you to be on time today because I can't wait for you two to get here! I must leave by half past seven or else I will miss my flight!'

'Sally, it'll be OK.'

'It won't be OK, Penny, because as I have reminded you numerous times in the past week, the nurse won't be able to come before ten o'clock today, and since you now won't be here by half past seven as planned it, Charlie will be home alone!'

'We are only running only thirty minutes late. She'll be fine, don't worry!'

'Never mind, it's pointless trying to make you understand because you never will do. Now, the nurse is coming at ten but if you will need to get hold of her for any reason, don't hesitate, just call her. I have written her phone number on the blackboard by the fridge in the kitchen. I have also written the doctor's cellular, home, and office number. And my neighbour's home and cellular numbers. If for any reason you need help, or simply have a question, don't hesitate to call any of them! I think I have covered everything. Well, one more thing. I will leave my house keys with my neighbour, Gary, so when you'll get here, buzz him and he will give you the keys. This is all for now so if you don't have any questions for me I will go.'

'I have no more questions so have a safe flight and see you later,' Penny says and they both hang up.

After about one and half hour of driving I pull over at Sally's place and park the car. Then, as instructed by Sally we knock at Gary's door who promptly hand us the keys. When we open Sally's front door we abandon our luggage by the front door and run downstairs.

Here there are three rooms: there is Charlie's room, the guest room, and the bathroom. Charlie's room is the biggest of all. It looks like a room one can expect to see in a hospital, immaculately clean and bright white, yet it is beautiful and cosy: there are fresh bouquets of red, white and yellow roses scattered all over the room. Around Charlie's bed there are just as many colourful vases with scented lilies and daises that successfully camouflage the true nature of the machines that are keeping Charlie alive. And then there is Charlie. She is lying in bed and watching the world going by with her eyes shut. She looks serene and painless, despite the tube coming out of her throat and all the needles puncturing her soft and delicate skin.

'Hi Charlie! Sorry we are late,' Penny says, kissing Charlie on her forehead and then moving slightly on the side to let me kiss her.

'Hi Charlie! If only either of you would merely spills the beans on how I can possibly make myself spring out of bed without having to push the snooze button over and over, I would never be late ever again! But let us not spoil this day we've anticipated so much with this matter now. How do you feel Charlie? Excited? Well, so do we!'

'Lilly, do you really think that she can hear you? I mean...'

'I know what you mean, Penny, and most likely she can't, but in doubt I talk to her! Besides, can you imagine how long it would take us to tell her all that she has missed while sleeping in the last three years?'

'Lilly, why are you still hoping for the impossible to happen? The doctors have clearly told us that she will never come out of her coma. Why are you deluding yourself into believing that she will?'

'I don't know, Penny, I guess for the same reason why you send her postcards from every place you go. Listen, if you take our luggage from upstairs and bring them here, I will start moving some furniture around and make room for the big screen. We really need to get going.'

'Very well, I'll switch the laptop on first and then I'll go.'

'Penny, why do you send her postcards?'

'I don't know, Lilly, I guess ... I guess it's my way of telling her that she's always with me everywhere I go ... I'm going upstairs to get the luggage.'

When Penny comes back she opens the cases and takes out the video projector and some cables and begins to connect the projector to the laptop.

'And why do you talk to her?'

'Somehow it helps me cope with the situation. The thought of coming here and telling her what has happened in our lives or reading her books keeps me going.'

'Can you pass me the blue cable, please?'

'The invitation expired an hour ago. Should we log in Facebook and see how many people have singed up for the event?'

'I don't think it's a good idea. Let's just wait and see, Lilly.'

'Why? Are you scared that no one would show up?'

'Well, not really, tho it'd be nice if they would. Can you turn on the projector, please?'

'Penny, we shouldn't feel any less proud of ourselves if people won't show up. Good, the projector works.'

'Certainly not, but if no one will show up, it means that we can't convey our message because nobody read our book. Let's assemble the projector screen now ... can you take all the pieces from the black suite case and put them on the floor over here please?'

'Sure, here they are ... I think that we are working ourselves up way too much over this! Just because people won't come for the signing and reading of our book, it doesn't necessarily mean that they haven't read it. Besides, sure that we want to inspire as many people as possible with our book, but it will be just as successful and rewarding if we can inspire only one.'

'Let's put the screen against that wall ... we better call the nurse, we are running out of time. Well I guess I could brush Charlie's hair if it comes down to it.'

'Don't need to do that my dear, I'm here now,' Annabel says while rushing into the room. '

'Hello Annabel! So good to see you! We don't have much time left. Do you think you can get Charlie ready in twenty minutes? Actually I can help you.

All we have left to do is to connect the projector with the Internet and since I'm a complete ignoramus when it comes to technology, I better leave Penny to it and let her work in peace.'

'It's actually a very good idea. Let's see...while I give her a sponge bath, you could trim her nails and brush her hair.'

'Very well!'

'There she is girls!' Penny shouts. 'Sally is online!'

'Hi Sally!' both Penny and I shout.

'Wait! The sound is off, she can't hear us! There we go. Try now.'

'Hi Sally! Can you hear us?' I ask.

'I can hear you loud and clear! Hello girls! How is everything going? Are you ready to go online in fifteen minutes?'

'We are ready, Sally!' Penny says.

'Very well! Girls, you'll have only ten minutes before you will be cut off, so make the most of your time! Now I have to go, they are opening the doors. I will talk to you in fifteen! Good luck!' Sally says before going offline.

They quickly get Charlie ready and put some make-up on. When they have finished they go standing by Charlie's bed and wait for Sally to come online.

Shortly after the big screen comes alive. Sally can be seen sitting behind a desk. A dozen girls are standing by her, looking right at Charlie, Penny and me, and more people are coming and joining them.

Sally is speaking to the audience.

'As promised, here are the authors of the book: Charlie, Lilly and Penny! Hello everyone! How are you?' Sally asks us.

'Hi everybody!' Penny and I say.

'These people have come here to meet you. What is your name, darling?' Sally asks one of the women standing by her. But the woman is staring at the projector screen and doesn't answer. So Sally asks her the question again and the girl resumes speaking.

'I ... I had no idea Charlie really existed. Is she the same Charlie the book talks about?'

'She is my dear, and so are Lilly and I!' Penny replies.

'Are the facts you've told in the book real then?' another girl in the audience asks in disbelief.

'They are all real hun, just as we all are indeed,' Penny proudly says.

'If any of you have any questions for Penny and Lilly, this is the time to do it!' Sally says as she looks at the group of people standing before her.

But no one in the audience say a word. They all look stunned. Sally is visibly uncomfortable and wordless, just as Penny and I are.

Finally one girl takes the stand and breaks the ice.

'After what happened to Charlie, is the airline doing anything to better the conditions of air stewardesses?' one girl in the crowd asks.

'Lilly, in the book you don't say what you do for a living, what do you do?' Another girl asks.

'And what did you two do after you found out what had happened to Charlie?' another girl in the very back asks.

'Please one question at a time,' Sally says. 'Let's start with you. What's your name?'

'Hi Lilly. My name is Tracy. At the end you decided to give up on becoming an air hostess. Looking back, do you regret it? I mean, with all due respect there are happy, glamorous air hostesses bouncing about the world and walking up and down the cabin. They surely don't look miserable or wanting to give up their job for anything else. Also, have you realised your dream to become a psychologist?'

'My dream came true, and I am indeed a psychologist. Funnily enough most of my clients are cabin crew members! Regarding your other question ... well, I don't regret it. First, I'm very happy to be doing what I do. Second, just as Penny and Charlie have said, cabin crew is not a career choice any more, and the only way one can truly enjoy it and be happy is by working part time or having a partner with a real job. Well, I was looking for a career, and I certainly wasn't looking to work part time. So to answer your question, no I don't regret it. Maybe in twenty years' time I will give it another shot, but not now.'

'Hi girls, my name is Lisa. I'm curious, where do you all live?' a girl asks.

'Shortly after having learned what had happened to Charlie, Penny and I decided to move to France, where Charlie and Sally were living.'

'Do you all live together then?' Lisa asks.

'No we don't. Lilly and I live in Paris, not far from each other, and Sally and Charlie live in Le Havre, in a beautiful house we all bought using most of the money my grandmother had left me.' says Penny.

'What about Charlie's family? Have they moved to Le Havre too?' another girl asks.

'Sadly enough,' Sally replies, 'when her parents learned what had happened to Charlie, they didn't want to take any part in it because as far as they were concerned, Charlie had called her misfortune upon herself. "She has always done whatever she wanted in her life," her mother told me, "and never once listened to us. So now you take care of her!" So I did from the very beginning, and we all do now.

'Why did it take you so long, Penny, to leave flying when you knew how unhealthy and ill you had become?' one girl asks.

'I hoped someone would ask me this question. I didn't have anything else to fall into, and lacking confidence in myself didn't make it any easier. But Charlie changed all that. She encouraged me to finally take action and get to grips with my life. For a long time I hid myself behind thousands of excuses that only contributed in the building of the spider's web that I ultimately fell victim to. I was constantly looking down on myself, and thinking how I wasn't good enough to do anything else but flying. I was restlessly looking for reasons to feel insecure and desperately trying to find ways to overcome it. Only after Charlie had given me the ultimatum, did I realise that finding the reasons why I was insecure was exactly what had prevented me from moving on. Just as Lilly told me once, not everything must have a reason, you just do it, you just move on. And that's exactly what I did.

'I didn't exactly know what I was going to do, but whatever it was, I was determined to do it. I searched the programmes the university was offering and merely chose one: beauty practitioner. I enrolled immediately and changed my life accordingly: applied for part-time, moved to a cheaper accommodation, sold my car, and dedicated most of my time to study. Before I knew it, I had a diploma in my hands, a job offer, and a way out from flying.'

'Have you come to terms with what happened to Charlie?' a girl asks.

'That's a very good question,' Penny says. 'I don't think we will ever do, and I'm sure I'm speaking on behalf of all of us, as we all are still carrying a great deal of guilt on our shoulders. There's not a day goes by that I don't regret not having reached out to Charlie when I had the chance to do it. Nothing and no one will ever bring Charlie back. We will never be able to rewind the time and do things differently.

However, what we can do is to learn from our mistakes and do whatever it takes to prevent them from happening again.

'And that's exactly what we did. What happened to Charlie can happen to anyone, because feeling trapped by one's fears can make us all vulnerable. Sally and I have been lucky enough to turn our lives round just in time, whereas Charlie didn't, and ultimately her feeling of guilt and fear prevailed against her potential to do something about them, ergo move on in life. When she realised it, unfortunately it was too late.

'Nevertheless, there is a valuable lesson to be learned and this is why we decided to write our stories: no one should ever give up on their dreams and more so on living happily ever after. Whether you think that there's no way out from a job you absolutely detest or your partner is making you feel horrible about yourself, there is indeed always a way out, just believe you can change your life and you will!'

'Besides, if you don't,' I jump in, 'you will not only make your life miserable but also everybody else's too, just as air hostess Ruth did to me on my way to Rome!'

'Or a bank employee did to me a few days ago,' Penny adds, 'who insulted me when I simply asked him if I could borrow his pen to sign the receipt he had handed to me?'

'Or a waiter rolled his eyes at me,' Sally jumps in, 'when I asked him politely to bring me some extra bread to the table.'

'Or a bus driver asked me in an annoyed manner if I knew where I was going when I merely asked him if he turned right at the traffic light,' I add.

'We only have one shot at this life, let's not waste it being miserable!' Penny speaks up. 'It's not doing you any good or anybody else you come in contact with for that matter!'

'The time is up,' Sally says. 'Thank you very much, girls!'

As soon as the crowd thank us and say goodbye, the big

projector turns black.

'It went better than expected!' I say.

'Too bad we didn't have time to share our delicious cake with them!' Penny says, going upstairs to get the cake.

'There is no cake,' I mumble.

'What? Don't tell me you forgot to bring the cake!'

'I did.'

'How could you? I repeatedly reminded you about it and even told you to stick a note on your front door! I bet you didn't do it, did you? Otherwise you would have remembered to bring it!'

'I did but I was running late and didn't pay attention to my note. I'll go to the store and buy one later. I know of a place in town where they make the best cakes! Now take a chair and come sit next to me. It's time to open our gifts.'

'You always manage to get away with everything! The least you can do then, is to buy the cake I like: a blackberry cobbler!'

'Fair enough! Now come here, my dear.'

I take a package from inside my hand bag and unwrap it.

'Happy birthday, Charlie!' I say.

'What book is it?' Penny asks.

'It's the *Cathedral of the Sea* by Ildefonso Falcones. I've read it a few years ago and I couldn't put it down!' I say. 'I'm sure Charlie will love it too.'

Penny says nothing and takes her gift from her handbag. She unwraps it.

'I kid you not, Lilly: it's the same book! I couldn't put it down either so I thought that Charlie wouldn't either!' Penny says.

'What are we waiting for? Let's dive into it! Charlie is becoming ever more anxious! Since I forgot to bring the cake, to you the honour to start reading this time.'

'We can read her a chapter each so we can go on all night long reading and put the book down only when it's finished!'

'Then you go and buy the cake now!' Penny quickly says.

'I'll go!' Annabel jumps in, 'so you girls can start reading to Charlie. She's indeed becoming anxious for you to start!'

Penny opens the book and starts to read:

'*Bernat realized nobody was looking in his direction, and glanced up at the clear blue sky…*'

EPILOGUE

It is time now to end my journey into the myth of cabin crew happily bouncing about the world in a cute uniform.

The inspiration to write about our lifestyle came when I realised how easy it is to fall for it and how hard it is to fall away from it with devastating consequences. Needless to say, the majority of people choose this 'career' for the wrong reasons, because they are driven by the assumption that being an air stewardess is still an idyllic job – which indeed it was in the 1970s and '80s when flying was expensive and was still largely the domain of executive businessmen. But as you well know by now, this is no longer the case.

As daunting and hard to accept as it is for many people who idealise this job, the truth is that nowadays cabin crew are challenged by ever more demanding passengers and competitive airlines that are constantly fighting to stay alive by taking cost-cutting measures. As a result it all comes down to this: cabin crew are now faced with low pay, a massive workload and long hours, which are unbearable for anyone's health, just as it had become for Penny, Charlie and me. Having said this, I hope inspired cabin crew can now make an informed decision on whether or not to go into this path, knowing exactly what they are getting into.

Furthermore, although what inspired me to write this book was our poisoned lifestyle, nevertheless I felt just as driven when I realised how one's life can be affected when feeling trapped into doing something one absolutely detests. In this respect, Charlie, Penny and myself are no different from anybody else who might happen to feel trapped in a career they wish to change or a relationship they wish to end. The truth is that no matter how impossible it might seem to turn one's own life around, it can be done just as I did, by following my dream, and as Penny did by embracing a new career and going for it.

Whether or not you believe in dancing, spinning and twirling dreams, it doesn't matter. Just start writing down your future and seal it in your red envelope!

www.ingramcontent.com/pod-product-compliance
Lightning Source LLC
Chambersburg PA
CBHW051248170626
46809CB00004B/1547